# The caregiver

# and

# the disabled child

*MARTIN STERLING*

## Table of contents

« *Accompanying a child with a disability is much more than providing medical care. It's about becoming his ally, understanding his silent needs, and offering him a space where every little progress is a victory. For the caregiver, it's a daily commitment to restoring dignity through simple gestures filled with humanity.* »

# 1.Introduction

# The role of the caregiver with disabled children

- **The changing landscape of care for disabled children**

The changing landscape of care for children with disabilities is marked by medical, social and legislative advances that have profoundly transformed the way these children are cared for. In the past, children with disabilities were often marginalized, their specific needs misunderstood or even ignored. They were often placed in isolated institutions where care was limited to purely medical aspects, often to the detriment of their psychological and social well-being.

Over the decades, a progressive awareness has emerged around the fact that these children have complex needs that cannot be reduced to a medical dimension. Society began to recognize their fundamental right to a life of dignity and fulfillment, with the same opportunities as any other child. This has led to a more holistic approach to care, integrating medical care, educational support and social accompaniment. One of the major turning points in this evolution has been the adoption of legislative frameworks such as the 2005 *Handicap Law* in France, which established a right to compensation for people with disabilities, including children, and placed the emphasis on school inclusion.

On the medical front, technological advances and advances in rehabilitation have significantly improved the quality of life for these children. Devices such as adapted wheelchairs and orthoses, as well as technological communication aids such as pictogram-based tablets, have transformed the daily lives of many non-verbal or mobility-impaired children. These innovations enable us to better respond to their specific needs, while promoting their autonomy.

The role of healthcare professionals, including nurses' aides, has also evolved. Whereas they were once seen as mere care providers, today they are recognized as essential players in the overall support of the child. They need to master a wide range of skills, from managing body care to adapting environments and communicating with children who are often unable to express themselves verbally. The relationship they forge with children becomes a vector of care in its own right, where listening and patience are tools as important as medical techniques.

Nurses now work in close collaboration with multidisciplinary teams, including nurses, specialized educators, psychologists and occupational therapists. This cooperation is crucial to developing individualized care plans that take into account not only the child's medical needs, but also his or her psychological, social and educational development. This multi-disciplinary approach fosters integrated care, with each professional bringing complementary expertise to bear on the child's life journey.

In addition, increased awareness of the rights of children with disabilities has reaffirmed their place in society. School inclusion, while still a challenge, has enabled many children to integrate into mainstream classes, with appropriate support. This inclusion is not only beneficial for the disabled child, but also for his or her peers, who learn to live with difference and develop an attitude of solidarity and respect.

Last but not least, changing attitudes have led to greater recognition and appreciation of the role played by families in the treatment process. Parents are no longer seen as mere observers, but as full partners in the therapeutic process. Their intimate knowledge of their child's needs makes them invaluable resources for healthcare professionals, and caregivers in particular must forge strong bonds of trust with them to ensure continuity and consistency in care.

As a result, the landscape of care for children with disabilities has evolved towards a more humane, inclusive and interdisciplinary approach, where the child is seen as a whole. This transformation has made it possible not only to improve living conditions for these children, but also to provide better support for families and change the collective mindset around disability. There is still progress to be made, but the foundations have now been laid to ensure that every child, whatever their condition, can receive the care and support they need to achieve their full potential.

- **Understanding the different types of disability in children**

Understanding the different types of disability in children is essential to providing appropriate, respectful and effective care. The term "disability" covers a wide variety of realities that impact a child's physical, intellectual, sensory or social development. Each type of disability presents specific challenges, but also unique strengths and potentialities that healthcare professionals, and especially caregivers, must learn to recognize in order to offer appropriate care.

Disabilities can be classified into several broad categories: motor disabilities, sensory disabilities, cognitive disabilities and neurodevelopmental disorders. Each of these categories encompasses a variety of situations that can vary in terms of severity and impact on the child's daily life.

Motor disabilities affect a child's mobility and ability to move, stand or perform everyday tasks. The causes can be varied: paralysis, neuromuscular diseases, congenital malformations or accidents. Cerebral palsy, for example, which results from early brain damage, is a frequent cause of motor disability in children. Depending on the severity of the injury, the child may need a wheelchair, orthoses or other technical aids to get around. For caregivers, this means adapting care and the environment to the child's physical capabilities, while ensuring maximum autonomy.

Sensory disabilities include impairments of hearing and sight. Deafness can range from a slight drop in hearing to total deafness, in which case the child may need to use hearing aids, lip-reading or sign language to communicate. Caregivers must therefore adapt their way of communicating, using visual aids, ensuring constant eye contact and creating an environment conducive to understanding. In the case of visually impaired or blind children, the visual impairment may limit their autonomy in everyday gestures, necessitating the use of white canes or assistive technologies such as voice-reading devices. Here again, the caregiver plays a key role in adjusting the child's care and activities to his or her visual capabilities, while promoting spatial orientation and safety.

Cognitive disabilities, also known as intellectual impairments, are characterized by significant limitations in intellectual functioning and coping skills, which manifest themselves before adulthood. These children may have difficulty understanding abstract concepts, solving problems or acquiring social and academic skills. Cognitive disabilities are often associated with conditions such as Down's syndrome, autism or global developmental delays. The intensity of these disabilities can vary considerably, with some children having a mild learning difficulty, while others may require constant support in most daily activities. For the caregiver, this means knowing how to use adapted teaching strategies, such as simplifying instructions, using images or objects to facilitate understanding, and above all, patience and repetition.

Neurodevelopmental disorders include conditions such as autism and attention deficit hyperactivity disorder (ADHD). Children with autism may have difficulty interacting socially, communicating verbally or non-verbally, and may also exhibit repetitive behaviors or restricted interests. These children may also be hypersensitive to certain sensory stimuli such as noise, light or touch. The caregiver must therefore be particularly attentive to these sensitivities, and take care to create a calm, predictable environment to avoid overloading the child. In the case of children with ADHD, difficulty in staying focused, impulsivity and hyperactivity call for appropriate care, where relaxation techniques and motor activities can help channel their energy.

It's important to note that some children may have multiple disabilities, i.e. a combination of several impairments (for example, an intellectual disability combined with motor or sensory disorders). These complex situations require even more individualized care, with particular attention paid to assessing each specific need and coordinating the various forms of care.

Beyond the categories of disability, it's crucial to remember that every child is unique. The same diagnosis can have very different consequences from one child to another, depending on his or her family environment, the quality of his or her support, and his or her own personal resources. As a caregiver, it is therefore essential to adopt a person-centred approach, taking the time to get to know the child, observe his or her reactions, listen to his or her needs, and involve parents or relatives in care decisions.

Finally, it's important to stress that disability should never be reduced to a limitation. Children with disabilities often have unsuspected strengths, be they creative abilities, perseverance, or a particular ability to connect with others on an emotional level. The role of the caregiver is to value these strengths, to encourage and participate in their development. This enables the child to grow up in an environment where he or she feels understood, supported and, above all, respected in his or her uniqueness.

- **The caregiver's specific role in the multidisciplinary team**

The caregiver's role in the multidisciplinary team is essential and unique, as he or she occupies a privileged position of proximity to the disabled child. Although often perceived as a support to nursing care, the caregiver plays a much broader, integrated role within the team. Working in collaboration with professionals such as nurses, doctors, psychologists, specialized educators and physiotherapists, the caregiver contributes to the development and implementation of adapted care, centered on the child's needs.

One of the caregiver's first responsibilities in this team dynamic is to provide basic care for the child, meeting daily needs such as hygiene, nutrition and comfort. This physical proximity enables the caregiver to build up a relationship of trust with the child, a relationship that becomes a real pillar of overall care. Thanks to this proximity, the caregiver can observe the child's day-to-day development, his reactions to care, his progress or his difficulties. They therefore play a watchful, observational role, essential for relaying relevant information to other team members. His daily observations, though sometimes perceived as simple, are in fact invaluable in adjusting care protocols or refining therapeutic strategies.

By being in direct contact with the child, the caregiver also becomes an important source of emotional support. Children with disabilities, whether they have physical, cognitive or sensory limitations, can experience frustration, anxiety or moments of distress. At such times, the caregiver is often the first person to offer comfort, through a caring presence, a gentle gesture or a soothing word. This role of emotional support, though subtle, has a major impact on the child's well-being, as it helps to create a climate of emotional security, conducive to his or her growth and development.

In addition to this relational dimension, the caregiver is involved in adapting the child's care environment. Working in close collaboration with other professionals, they help to create an environment adapted to the specific needs of each child. For example, in the case of a child with motor difficulties, he or she ensures that the environment is accessible and safe, and that equipment is positioned to facilitate movement and handling. Similarly, for a child with sensory difficulties, the caregiver may suggest adjustments to reduce disruptive sensory stimuli, such as soft lighting or a reduction in surrounding noise.

One of the caregiver's most important roles in the multidisciplinary team is that of coordinating basic care with specialized interventions. For example, during a rehabilitation program with a physiotherapist, the caregiver may be called upon to continue certain exercises on a daily basis, thus integrating mobilization or posture activities into routine care. They also ensure that the recommendations made by speech therapists or occupational therapists are followed during meals and playtime. This continuity of care, ensured by the caregiver, is crucial to guaranteeing the effectiveness of specialized interventions and maximizing the child's well-being.

The caregiver must also work closely with the child's family, who play a central role in the care provided. They often act as a link between the professionals and the parents, explaining the care provided, reassuring them about the child's progress, and offering practical advice on how to continue the care at home. This partnership relationship is essential to ensure consistency between the care given in the facility and that given to the child, which is particularly important in long or complex cases.

The multidisciplinary team also relies on the ability of each professional to exchange information smoothly and efficiently. In this respect, the caregiver plays a key role in transmitting information about the child's condition. Whether at coordination meetings, or during transmissions at the beginning or end of the day, they must communicate their observations accurately and factually to other team members. These exchanges make it possible to adjust care plans, modify certain therapeutic approaches, or plan additional interventions if necessary. The caregiver thus becomes an indispensable cog in the team's communication chain.

Beyond the technical aspect, the caregiver must also be able to integrate an ethical dimension into his or her work within the multidisciplinary team. Working with disabled children raises complex ethical issues, such as respect for the child's dignity and right to autonomy, and managing consent when the child is unable to express him/herself. In these situations, the caregiver's role as a close companion often involves mediating between the team and the family, while ensuring that the child's fundamental rights are respected.

- **The essential skills of the caregiver: listening, empathy and patience**

Caregivers' essential skills, such as listening, empathy and patience, are at the heart of the quality of the care they provide, especially when accompanying children with disabilities. These human qualities, although they may seem obvious, are in fact crucial professional skills, as they shape not only the relationship with the child, but also with his or her family and the care team.

**Listening** is undoubtedly one of the most fundamental skills for a caregiver. In the context of disability, where children may have difficulty communicating verbally or expressing their needs, listening goes far beyond words. It involves knowing how to observe and understand non-verbal signs, behaviors or physical reactions that reveal the child's emotional state or immediate need. For example, a non-verbal child may express discomfort through moaning or agitated behavior. The caregiver must be attentive to these signals and be able to interpret them to respond appropriately to the child's needs.

This ability to listen is not limited to the child, but also extends to the family. Parents of children with disabilities, often faced with daily challenges and deep-seated anxieties, may express their worries or fatigue through words or behavior. The caregiver must be able to actively listen to these concerns without judgment, understand them in all their complexity and respond with kindness. This quality of listening not only helps to build trusting relationships with families, but also contributes to improving the child's overall care, as parents become full partners in the care process.

**Empathy** is one of the most valuable human skills in the field of care, and it is particularly essential for the caregiver. Empathy is the ability to put oneself in another person's shoes, to feel what they're feeling, while maintaining a professional distance that enables them to act appropriately. When working with disabled children, the caregiver must constantly show empathy to understand the frustrations, pains or difficulties the child may encounter in his or her daily life. This can manifest itself in simple gestures, such as adapting one's work rhythm to that of the child, giving him or her more time to complete a task, or simply being present at moments when the child expresses anxiety.

Empathy is also essential in recognizing that each child has a unique experience. A child with a physical disability may feel frustrated by his or her limitations, while a child with sensory difficulties may experience anxiety in over-stimulating environments. The caregiver must understand these realities, adapt his or her approach and offer personalized support to each individual. This ability to understand the other person's emotions and needs, without being overwhelmed by them, creates a climate of care where the child feels safe, understood and respected.

Empathy is just as important when dealing with families. Parents of disabled children may be confronted with feelings of guilt, sadness or exhaustion. The caregiver must be able to recognize these emotions, welcome them and support the parents without minimizing their feelings. For example, when parents express concern about their child's future, it's crucial to listen with empathy, offer emotional support and, if necessary, refer them to appropriate resources. Empathy enables the caregiver to reinforce this relationship of trust with families, which is essential for harmonious care.

Finally, **patience** is a skill that underpins all the others, and is absolutely essential in the caregiver's day-to-day work. Caring for children with disabilities often means repeating gestures, instructions or activities, with no guarantee of immediate results. Whether for simple tasks such as helping a child get dressed, or more complex situations such as managing a crisis, patience is essential. The caregiver must accept that progress is sometimes slow, and that each child evolves at his or her own pace.

This patience is particularly crucial when communicating with children who have difficulty expressing themselves. It can be tempting, when faced with a child who doesn't react or doesn't seem to understand, to want to go faster or repeat instructions. However, a patient caregiver will adapt his or her language, rephrase instructions and give the child the time he or she needs to react. This is all the more important as some children may need regular breaks or more time to process information. This approach, which respects children's rhythms, contributes to their well-being and development.

Patience is also needed to manage moments of crisis or frustration. Children with disabilities can sometimes express their distress through unmanageable behavior, such as agitation or aggression. The caregiver must demonstrate great self-control and patience to defuse these situations without rushing the child, while maintaining a secure and reassuring environment. Patience, in these moments, is synonymous with control, benevolence and respect.

# 2.

# Welcoming and accompanying disabled children

- **Welcoming children and their families: building a relationship of trust**

Welcoming the child and his or her family is a fundamental moment in the care of children with disabilities. It is at this precise moment that the foundation of a relationship of trust is laid, which will condition the quality of care and well-being of the child throughout his or her life. This reception is not just a simple administrative formality or a series of medical assessments. It is a delicate and humane process, in which the caregiver plays a central role in ensuring that the child and his or her family feel listened to, respected and safe.

The first meeting with a child and his or her family is often emotionally charged. For parents, entrusting their child to professionals can be a source of anxiety, fear and sometimes guilt. They often arrive with both expectations and fears, faced with the unknown and the possible trials that await them. Some parents may have had difficult experiences with the healthcare system in the past, adding to their apprehension. This is why the welcome must be marked by kindness and sensitivity. The caregiver, through his or her posture, gestures and words, has the ability to reassure and show that each member of the family, and especially the child, will be taken into account in all his or her uniqueness.

**Creating a relationship of trust** begins with active listening. From the very first minutes, the caregiver must offer the family a space to express their needs, questions and concerns. It's crucial not to interrupt them, or minimize their concerns, but rather to welcome them with empathy. The caregiver's attentive listening, often non-verbal through nods or soothing smiles, conveys an essential message: "We're here for you, we understand you." This active listening must also extend to the child, even if he or she is non-verbal or has difficulty expressing him or herself. The caregiver must be attentive to the child's body language, facial expressions or gestures, and show the child that he or she is just as important as his or her parents.

**Empathy** is also a key component of this welcome. The parents of a disabled child often experience moments of great vulnerability. They may feel overwhelmed by their child's needs, or saddened by unfulfilled expectations. By acknowledging these emotions and welcoming them without judgment, the caregiver helps to strengthen the relationship of trust. Saying to a parent "I understand how difficult this must be for you", or simply being present during a moment of strong emotion, shows the family that the caregiver is there not only to care for the child, but also to support them in their journey.

In addition to listening and empathy, **transparency** is another essential pillar in building trust. Parents often need to know exactly what is going to happen to their child, whether in terms of care, interventions or long-term goals. The caregiver must provide clear, accessible and honest information about the care process. The aim is not to hide any difficulties or uncertainties, but to address them with sincerity. Explaining the stages of the care process, detailing the procedures that will be carried out, or answering parents' questions in a transparent way, reinforces their sense of security. When parents feel they have been fully informed, they are more likely to trust the healthcare team and become actively involved in their child's care.

**Respect for the child** in this process is just as fundamental. From the very outset, it's important to consider the child as a person in his or her own right, with his or her own needs, fears and desires. This means including them in discussions as much as possible, and explaining to them what is going to happen, even if they are very young or have a severe disability. Asking him if he agrees before touching him, showing him medical instruments before using them, or speaking softly to him, are simple gestures that show the child that he is respected and listened to. This respect helps to create an environment in which the child feels secure, fostering greater cooperation in care and a calmer relationship with the nursing team.

Finally, welcoming the child and his or her family is also a time when the caregiver **takes the time to understand family dynamics**. Every family is unique, and the relationships between parents and children, or between different family members, can influence the way the child reacts to care. The caregiver must be sensitive to these dynamics, while respecting the family's culture, values and beliefs. In some families, for example, caring for a disabled child may give rise to tensions or misunderstandings. By paying attention to these elements and engaging in respectful dialogue, the caregiver can help defuse certain difficulties and strengthen cohesion around the child's care.

- **First contact with the child: assessing specific needs**

The first contact with a disabled child is a key stage in assessing his or her specific needs and laying the foundations for appropriate care. It's a delicate moment, because it's not simply a matter of gathering medical information or carrying out a technical assessment, but of gaining an in-depth understanding of the child in all his or her uniqueness: his or her abilities, limitations, preferences and modes of communication. The caregiver plays an essential role here, as he or she is often one of the first contacts with the child and his or her family, and this first contact determines the quality of future care.

During this first meeting, one of the first aspects to consider **is careful observation of the child**. Children with disabilities can often have difficulty expressing their needs or feelings verbally, especially in the presence of a new environment or unfamiliar people. The caregiver must therefore be attentive to the child's behavior, facial expressions, movements and body language. These elements can give valuable clues as to how the child is feeling: is he anxious? Does he feel confident? Is he in physical pain? Every gesture, every expression can reveal clues to the child's physical or emotional state of health.

Observation is all the more important as it enables us to **detect the** child's **modes of communication**. Some children, particularly those with autism spectrum disorders or intellectual disabilities, may use non-verbal means to communicate. The caregiver must be able to identify these means, be they gestures, signs or looks. The child may also use assisted communication tools, such as pictograms or digital tablets, to express his or her needs. In this case, it is important to ask the family or professionals who know the child to explain how these tools are used, so that they can be integrated into daily care.

**Understanding the child's specific disability** is another crucial aspect of this initial assessment. Every child has particular needs depending on his or her disability, and it's essential to take the time to fully understand the characteristics of his or her condition. For example, a child with cerebral palsy may have specific needs in terms of mobility, positioning or comfort, while a child with a sensory impairment will require an environment adapted to his or her hearing or visual limitations. Understanding disability also means finding out about any equipment the child uses, such as orthoses, wheelchairs or hearing aids, and how these tools facilitate his or her daily life.

The caregiver should also **involve the parents or guardians** in this initial assessment. Parents are their child's first experts. They know their child's reactions, habits, preferences and needs better than anyone else. During this first meeting, the caregiver should therefore adopt an active listening attitude, asking open-ended questions that will enable the parents to share all relevant information. For example, it may be useful to ask: "How does your child react to new environments?" or "Are there things that particularly soothe him when he's anxious?". This dialogue not only provides practical information, but also builds a relationship of trust with parents, who then feel respected and listened to in their knowledge of their child.

Alongside this information gathering, the caregiver needs to pay particular attention **to** the child's **immediate environment**.

During the first contact, it may be necessary to observe how the child interacts with the space around him. Does he feel comfortable in a bright room, or does he need a quieter, more subdued environment? Is he able to move around on his own, or does he need help? Does he need a safe space where he can move freely without the risk of falling or injuring himself? By observing these interactions, we can begin to adapt the environment to the child's specific needs, whether this involves rearranging furniture or reducing visual and sound stimuli.

Another essential aspect of the first contact is **the assessment of medical and therapeutic needs**. This involves identifying current treatments, any medication the child is taking and any specific care he or she may require. For example, a child with swallowing difficulties may need adapted feeding or specific techniques to be fed safely. In this context, the caregiver must not only find out about these needs, but also ensure that the appropriate medical protocols are in place and known to all members of the multidisciplinary team.

However, assessing a child's specific needs is not limited to a medical or technical approach. **The emotional and psychological aspect** is just as important. During initial contact, the caregiver should pay close attention to the child's emotional state, observing his or her reactions to strangers or new situations. Some children may be very anxious or resistant, while others are more at ease. In all cases, it's important to offer the child a reassuring environment, explaining (even if he doesn't seem to understand verbally) what's going to happen, taking the time to reassure him with gentle gestures, and giving him time to adapt. Establishing an initial soothing and reassuring relationship helps to lay a solid foundation for further care.

Finally, it's important to remember that this first contact must be made with **great cultural and family sensitivity**. Each family has its own way of understanding disability and caring for its child. The caregiver must be attentive to cultural or religious particularities that may influence care. For example, some families may have specific preferences in terms of food, clothing or social interaction. Respecting these elements from the very first contact helps to create a relationship of mutual respect, while ensuring that care is in line with the family's values and beliefs.

- **The importance of individualized care**

The importance of individualized care is paramount in the care of children with disabilities. Every child is unique, with his or her own needs, abilities and limitations. Disability, whether physical, sensory or cognitive, does not manifest itself in the same way in all children, even when they share a similar diagnosis. A standardized approach to care risks neglecting crucial aspects of the child's well-being, which is why individualized care is essential to ensure not only the child's physical health, but also his or her emotional and social development.

At the heart of individualized care **lies the recognition of each child's uniqueness**. A medical diagnosis, such as cerebral palsy, autism spectrum disorder or visual impairment, does not in itself define how a child should be cared for. Each child has a unique way of experiencing his or her disability, and this diversity must be taken into account when drawing up the care plan. For example, two children with autism may have totally different needs: one may be non-verbal and need support to communicate, while the other may be fluent but require special supervision to manage social interactions. Individualized care therefore enables us to **meet the specific needs of each child**, taking into account his or her strengths and weaknesses.

Personalized care begins with **an in-depth, ongoing assessment of the** child's needs. It is not enough to rely solely on a medical diagnosis; it is necessary to observe the child in different contexts to understand his or her functional abilities, reactions to the environment, preferences and difficulties. For example, a child with a motor impairment may be perfectly capable of carrying out certain activities, provided the equipment is adapted and gestures are facilitated. Personalizing care therefore means **implementing specific strategies**, such as the use of technical aids (wheelchairs, orthoses, etc.) or augmentative communication tools (pictograms, tablets). These devices, adapted to the child, enable him or her to overcome certain barriers and actively participate in daily life.

Individualized care also **means adapting the environment**. One of the most important aspects of this approach is the ability to adjust the space around the child to make it as conducive as possible to his or her well-being and autonomy. This can include modifications to the physical space (adapted furniture, subdued lighting for light-sensitive children, reduced noise stimuli for children with sensory disorders) or the design of specific routines that meet the child's needs. A child with behavioral problems linked to autism, for example, will benefit from a structured, predictable environment, where every activity is planned and announced in advance. This organization gives the child a sense of security and control, thus limiting the onset of anxiety attacks.

Individualized care not only concerns the physical and material aspects, but also **the relational aspects**. The way we interact with the child must also be adapted to his or her specific needs. Some disabled children may have difficulty making eye contact or maintaining a verbal conversation. Others may be more comfortable with gentle physical contact or encouraging gestures. The caregiver must be attentive to these signals and adapt his or her approach to respect the child's rhythm and mode of communication. For example, a non-verbal child may need more time to respond to a prompt, and the caregiver should allow this space without rushing or assuming that the child has not understood.

Flexibility is another essential component of individualized care. A child's needs may evolve over time, in line with his or her development or changes in health. A care strategy that works today may no longer be appropriate in a few months' time. It is therefore important for the caregiver, and the whole multidisciplinary team, to be able to adjust care based on new observations or feedback from parents. This flexibility implies regular assessment of the child's situation and ongoing communication with the family to ensure that care remains relevant and effective.

**Collaboration with parents** is a fundamental element of individualized care. Parents know their child better than anyone else, and are often the first to notice subtle changes in their child's behavior, needs or abilities. The caregiver needs to work hand-in-hand with them, valuing their knowledge and involving them in decisions about their child's care. This may include adjustments to the daily routine, adaptations to feeding, or changes in communication modalities. This collaborative approach ensures that the child benefits from consistent care, both at home and in care facilities, and that all dimensions of his or her well-being are taken into account.

Last but not least, individualized care is not just about meeting the child's immediate needs; it must also be aimed at **fostering the child's** long-term **autonomy and development**. It's not just a question of compensating for the limitations imposed by the disability, but of enabling the child to develop his or her own skills, gain autonomy and actively participate in his or her environment. This can take the form of rehabilitation programs, cognitive or sensory stimulation activities, or adapted leisure time. The aim is to enable the child, as far as possible, to develop, learn and interact with the world around him, despite the challenges imposed by his disability.

- **Preparing and adapting the care environment for each child**

Preparing and adapting the care environment for each child with a disability is an essential step in ensuring their well-being, meeting their specific needs and fostering their development. The care environment is not just limited to the physical layout of the premises; it also includes the emotional atmosphere, the quality of interactions, and the adaptation of routines. Each child, depending on his or her disability, abilities and sensitivity, reacts differently to the environment around him or her. Careful preparation and ongoing adaptation are therefore essential if this space is to become reassuring, stimulating and conducive to the child's overall being-well.

The first step in preparing the care environment is to **understand the child's sensory and physical needs**. Each disability has its own specificities, and the environment must be adapted accordingly. For example, a child with a motor impairment may need clear, easily accessible spaces to move around in a wheelchair or to use technical aids. Doors, furniture and even everyday objects need to be adjusted to allow the child to move around freely and, as far as possible, acquire a degree of autonomy. Accessibility is therefore a central criterion in the preparation of the space, to enable the child to feel at ease and participate actively in daily activities.

Similarly, for children with sensory impairments, **the environment must be designed to compensate for or minimize auditory or visual limitations**. For example, a visually impaired child will benefit from an environment with clear tactile or auditory cues, where important objects are predictably placed and accessible. Furniture can be color contrasted to help the child identify different elements, and potential obstacles should be avoided to reduce the risk of falls. For a deaf or hard-of-hearing child, it's important that room lights are well adjusted to facilitate lip-reading or the use of sign language. The introduction of visual systems, such as light signals to replace warning sounds, is also a common adaptation to better meet the child's specific needs.

**Managing sensory stimuli** is another fundamental element in preparing the care environment. Children with autism spectrum disorders, for example, are often highly sensitive to external stimuli such as loud noises, bright light or physical contact. For these children, it's essential to create a soothing environment, where stimuli are controlled and minimized. This can include the use of soft, subdued lighting, the reduction of ambient noise through soundproofing materials, or the installation of curtains to filter natural light. Similarly, certain rooms can be fitted out with sensory objects or safe spaces, where the child can retreat in the event of sensory overload. This type of environment, designed to soothe and secure the child, promotes emotional well-being and reduces the risk of anxiety attacks or agitation.

At the same time, **it**'s important to take **into account the child's preferences in terms of interaction and communication**. Some children, especially those with cognitive disorders or intellectual disabilities, may need a stable routine and structured environment to feel secure. The preparation of the care environment should therefore include visual cues, pictograms or pictorial calendars, which help the child to anticipate the different stages of the day. For example, the child may know that it's mealtime when a picture of breakfast is displayed, or understand that it's time to wash his hands when he sees a corresponding picture. This visual structuring of space and time helps children better understand their environment, and reduces uncertainty, a potential source of anxiety.

Adapting the care environment also includes **taking into account the emotional and relational aspects**. A care environment must not simply be a functional place where the child's physical needs are met; it must also be a reassuring and welcoming space, where the child feels safe and surrounded by kindness. To achieve this, it's important to personalize the space according to the child's tastes and preferences. If a child is particularly attached to a toy, a blanket or an object that comforts him, it's essential that this object is accessible in his daily environment. Small adjustments, such as displaying pictures or drawings that the child likes, can help to make the space more familiar and pleasant, and thus facilitate the child's adaptation to the care environment.

Family involvement in this preparation is also essential. **Parents are often the best guides** to help understand what works for their child. They know the child's habits and reactions to certain stimuli, and can provide valuable pointers on how the environment should be designed. Working closely with parents helps to create a space that reflects the child's real needs, not just those assumed by healthcare professionals. This collaboration also reinforces the coherence between the care environment and the home environment, facilitating the child's transition between these two spaces.

Finally, the adaptation of the care environment should not be fixed. **The child's needs evolve over time**, and it's important to regularly reassess the space to ensure that it remains suitable. This may involve adjusting to the child's changing abilities, introducing new equipment, or modifying certain elements to suit new preferences or sensitivities. The care environment must remain flexible and evolving, so that it continues to meet the child's needs optimally throughout his or her development.

# 3.

# Daily care: technical gestures and humanity

- **Basic care: hygiene, nutrition and comfort**

Basic care - hygiene, nutrition and comfort - is the foundation of daily care for children with disabilities. Although this care may seem routine, it requires special attention, as each child has specific needs linked to his or her disability. Ensuring proper hygiene, providing a balanced diet and guaranteeing the child's physical and emotional comfort are actions that require not only technical skills, but also a deep sensitivity to each child's individual needs. This care is not limited to mechanical gestures: it involves a holistic and personalized approach, in which the child's overall well-being is constantly at the center of attention.

**Hygiene**, the first element of basic care, plays a fundamental role in a child's physical and psychological health. Children with disabilities, particularly those with motor or cognitive limitations, may find it difficult to maintain their personal hygiene independently. In such cases, the caregiver helps them with essential daily tasks, such as washing hands, brushing teeth, grooming and dressing. In some cases, these gestures must be performed entirely by the caregiver, while in others, the child can participate, even partially, in his or her own grooming. The aim is always to promote the child's autonomy, by accompanying and encouraging him/her to perform these tasks by him/herself wherever possible. Despite his limitations, the child should be encouraged to take an active part in these activities, as this not only helps to preserve his self-esteem, but also reinforces his motor and cognitive skills.

Body hygiene is also an ideal time for the caregiver to establish a bond of trust with the child. Hygiene care requires regular physical contact, which must be carried out with gentleness and respect. Some children, particularly those suffering from autism spectrum disorders or sensory sensitivity, may be reluctant to certain textures or sensations. The caregiver must therefore adapt to each child by respecting his or her preferences and creating a soothing environment. For example, a child may prefer water at a particular temperature, or need slower movements to feel secure.

By adapting care to individual needs, the caregiver transforms a potentially stressful act into a reassuring moment for the child.

**Nutrition**, the second pillar of basic care, is of vital importance to a child's development and health. Many children with disabilities have specific nutritional needs, due to chewing or swallowing difficulties, or metabolic disorders. Some children require dietary adaptations, such as blended meals or reducing the size of pieces to facilitate swallowing. Other children, particularly those with neurological disorders, can be fed via enteral feeding devices, such as a gastric tube. The caregiver must be particularly vigilant in the preparation and management of meals, taking care to respect the dietary recommendations established by the medical team.

But there's much more to food than just nutrition. Meals are also important social and emotional moments. For a child, eating in a calm, pleasant environment, in the company of adults or other children, can transform this moment into a positive experience. The caregiver must ensure that these moments are stress-free for the child, by adapting his or her work rhythm and respecting the child's particular needs. For example, it may be necessary to give a child more time to finish his meal, or to help him hold his cutlery so that he can participate actively. These moments are also an opportunity to reinforce the child's autonomy: even a child with motor difficulties can learn to use a spoon or drink on his own, with the right guidance and support.

**Comfort** is the third fundamental aspect of basic care. Ensuring a child's physical and emotional comfort is essential to prevent discomfort, pain or complications related to his or her disability. For a child with reduced mobility, physical comfort means regularly adjusting the child's position to avoid pressure sores or pain caused by muscular contractures. The caregiver must pay close attention to the way the child is positioned in the wheelchair or bed, ensuring that cushions or orthopedic supports are correctly positioned to optimize comfort. A poorly positioned child can quickly experience discomfort or develop pain, affecting not only mobility, but also mood and ability to participate in activities.

Emotional comfort is just as important as physical comfort. A child with a disability, especially in a care environment, may feel anxious, isolated or misunderstood. The caregiver plays a key role in creating an emotionally secure environment, where the child feels listened to, respected and supported. This involves a caring attitude and gentle, reassuring gestures, as well as adapting the environment to make it more welcoming. For example, some children may feel more at ease if they have familiar objects nearby, such as a favorite toy or a special blanket, to comfort and reassure them.

Attention to the child's comfort is not limited to the daytime; it also includes care during sleep. As sleep is crucial to the child's recovery and development, the caregiver must ensure that the child sleeps in good conditions, with a mattress adapted to his needs, and that his position is regularly changed to avoid any physical discomfort. Peaceful sleep and rest are essential if the child is to face the day with greater serenity and well-being.

- **Adapting care to motor, sensory or cognitive disabilities**

Adapting care to motor, sensory or cognitive impairments is essential to providing respectful and effective care for children with disabilities. Each type of disability presents specific challenges that require an individualized approach. The caregiver must be able to adjust not only technical gestures, but also the environment and interaction with the child, to guarantee his or her well-being, comfort and development. This ability to is adapt the fruit of careful observation, a deep understanding of the child's needs and great flexibility in care.

**Motor** ,disabilities whether of neurological, congenital or traumatic origin, affect a child's mobility and ability to perform certain actions independently. Some children may have partial or total paralysis, while others may suffer from coordination disorders or muscle spasticity. Adapting care in this context means first and foremost paying particular attention to the child's **positioning**. A child with motor difficulties may spend long hours in a sitting or lying position, and poor positioning can lead to pain, muscle contractures or bedsores. The caregiver must therefore ensure that the child is positioned comfortably and safely, using cushions, orthopedic supports or adapted wheelchairs to avoid any physical discomfort.

Accompanying children with motor disabilities also **means adapting daily activities**. For hygiene care, such as toileting, it may be necessary to use lifting devices to move the child safely, or to adapt the bathroom with support bars and specialized seats. Similarly, for meals, some children may need special utensils, such as thick-handled spoons or spill-proof cups, to enable them to eat or drink more independently. In all cases, the caregiver must take care to offer the child the opportunity to participate in care as much as possible, respecting his or her rhythm and abilities, and rewarding every little effort.

Care for children with motor disabilities also involves **rigorous prevention of complications associated with immobility**. Care must include massages to stimulate blood circulation, gentle passive mobilization exercises to prevent joint stiffness, and constant monitoring of areas at risk of bedsores. These gestures, although technical, are also privileged moments for creating a bond of trust with the child and ensuring his overall well-being.

For **sensory disabilities,** whether visual or auditory, the adaptation of care is based on the way in which the child communicates and interacts with her/him, as well as on the environment. A visually impaired or blind child may need detailed verbal support to understand what is going on around him. When providing care, it's essential to **verbalize every gesture** before carrying it out. For example, before starting a toilet, the caregiver can describe the various steps to come, explaining which product to use and where to touch it. This verbal anticipation helps the child to prepare mentally and feel secure. In addition, it is important to use tactile and auditory cues, such as specific objects or familiar sounds, to help the child orientate himself in his environment and better apprehend the care.

For deaf or hard-of-hearing children, **visual communication** becomes central. We need to adapt the way we communicate, using sign language if the child has mastered it, or reinforcing the use of gestures, mimics and pictograms. Eye contact is fundamental: the caregiver must ensure that the child looks at him/her when he/she speaks, so that he/she can read his/her lips or observe his/her facial expressions. It's also useful to establish clear, predictable routines, so that the child knows in advance what's going to happen, thus reducing anxiety linked to misunderstanding.

**In the case of cognitive disabilities,** such as intellectual disabilities or autism spectrum disorders, the adaptation of care must take into account the child's difficulties in understanding and interacting with his or her environment. Children with intellectual retardation or cognitive disorders may have difficulty following complex instructions or anticipating the steps involved in care. In such cases, a simplified, structured approach is essential. **Breaking tasks down into small steps**, using short, simple sentences, and repeating instructions consistently are effective strategies to help the child understand and participate in care. For example, when toileting, the caregiver can describe each action concisely: "Now wash your hands", "Rinse off the soap", "Dry off". Each step is accompanied by a visual demonstration or physical guidance to help the child follow along.

Children with cognitive disorders, especially those with autism, may also need a particularly **predictable and stable** environment. Sudden changes, loud noises or unexpected physical contact can cause stress and seizures. It is therefore important to establish regular routines and create a soothing environment with few disruptive stimuli. The caregiver must also be attentive to the **sensory particularities** of these children. Some may be hypersensitive to certain textures, temperatures or sounds, while others seek out specific stimuli. Adapting care to these sensitivities, for example by choosing care products with a particular texture or adjusting the lighting in the room, helps to make the care experience more pleasant for the child.

Supporting children with cognitive disabilities also involves **reinforcing social skills and communication**, even when the child has difficulty expressing himself verbally. Alternative communication tools, such as pictograms or electronic tablets, can be a great help in enabling the child to communicate his or her needs and feelings. Caregivers need to be trained in the use of these tools and know how to integrate them into daily care, so that the child can actively participate in his or her own care.

- **Managing pain and comfort in non-communicative children**

Managing pain and comfort in a non-communicative child is a major challenge for healthcare professionals, especially caregivers, as the child cannot verbalize his or her feelings or express directly what is bothering him or her. However, even without the use of speech, the child shows many signs of his condition, and the caregiver must know how to observe, interpret and act on these subtle clues to ensure adequate care. Pain management and the promotion of comfort in these children are not only essential for their physical well-being, but also for their emotional and psychological well-being.

**Observing and interpreting non-verbal signs of pain** is the first step in managing pain in non-communicative children. In the absence of verbal language, children express their pain through bodily behaviors, facial expressions, cries, groans or changes in attitude. A child in pain may, for example, stiffen up, rub a particular area of the body, curl up, or become agitated. Changes in eating or sleeping habits, as well as sudden or prolonged crying, are also valuable clues. The caregiver must be able to recognize these signs and relate them to any physical pain. It's important to get to know the child and establish a baseline of daily behavior, so you can quickly spot any deviations or unusual manifestations that might signal pain.

Another fundamental aspect in identifying pain in non-communicative children is **to pay attention to specific reactions during care**. Certain gestures, such as touching a particular area, changing position or even a simple touch, can trigger a pain reaction in the child. If the child reacts negatively to specific actions (for example, if he tenses up or cries when his arm or back is manipulated), this can be a clear sign of pain. It is then crucial for the caregiver to adapt his or her approach, handling the child with great gentleness and avoiding any manipulation that could aggravate the pain. What's more, once the care has been performed, it's essential to assess the effect of these gestures on the child's behavior: if he becomes calmer or more agitated, this gives an indication of the intensity of his pain and the comfort he feels.

**Behavioral pain assessment scales**, such as the FLACC (Face, Legs, Activity, Cry, Consolability) scale, are valuable tools for objectifying pain in non-communicative children. These scales record specific behaviors such as facial expressions, body movements and response to attempts at consolation. The caregiver, trained in the use of these tools, can thus regularly measure the intensity of the child's pain and adjust care accordingly, while alerting the rest of the care team if further medical management is required.

Alongside pain management, **ensuring the child's physical comfort** is just as important. For a non-communicative child, physical discomfort can quickly lead to agitation, stress and a deterioration in general condition. Comfort involves several aspects, not least the child's positioning. An immobile or immobile child can suffer from muscular pain, stiffness or pressure sores if not properly positioned. To avoid these complications, the caregiver must regularly reposition the child, using positioning cushions and anti-pressure-sore mattresses, and ensuring that the child is installed in a position that is both comfortable and secure.

**The care environment** also plays a key role in the child's comfort. An environment that is too noisy, too bright or too cold can be a source of stress and discomfort. The caregiver must therefore take care to create a soothing environment, with soft lighting, a pleasant temperature and few disruptive stimuli. Non-communicative children, especially those with sensory or cognitive disorders, can be very sensitive to their immediate environment. Careful adjustment of room conditions can help them to relax and improve their general comfort.

**The emotional dimension of comfort** should not be overlooked either. A non-communicative child may express emotional discomfort or distress through crying or agitation. As well as providing physical comfort, the caregiver must be attentive to the child's emotional needs. A reassuring presence, gentle physical contact such as holding the child's hand, or soothing words - even if the child doesn't understand the words - all help to create a secure environment. The caring and attentive attitude of the caregiver, who knows how to adapt his or her pace and gestures to the child's reactions, is essential in establishing a climate of trust and serenity.

**The use of non-medicinal techniques** to relieve pain and improve comfort is also very useful for non-communicative children. These techniques include gentle massage, thermotherapy (application of hot or cold compresses to certain areas of the body), controlled sensory stimulation or the use of soothing music. These methods reduce muscular tension, distract the child from pain or discomfort, and promote general relaxation. The caregiver must be trained in these techniques and able to apply them in a way that is adapted to the child's needs and reactions.

Finally, managing pain and comfort in a non-communicative child relies on **close collaboration with the family and other**

**healthcare professionals**. Parents often know best the subtle signs that their child is in pain or discomfort. Their observation and experience are valuable resources for the caregiver, who must work hand in hand with them to adjust care to the child's reactions. In addition, collaboration with the multidisciplinary team (nurses, doctors, physiotherapists) ensures comprehensive pain management, including, if necessary, drug treatments or specific interventions to improve the child's comfort.

- **Crisis care: calming and soothing the child**

Caring for a disabled child in a crisis situation demands special attention, as these moments are often marked by great emotional distress, frustration and even pain. Calming and soothing a child in crisis requires not only technical skills, but also a deep sensitivity and an approach adapted to the child's situation and personality. The caregiver, on the front line at these critical moments, plays an essential role by adopting a caring attitude, providing appropriate responses and creating a secure environment for the child. The aim is to defuse the crisis gently and progressively, while re-establishing a climate of calm and trust.

The first step in managing a crisis is to **understand what triggers it**. Children with disabilities, whether they have cognitive, sensory or motor disorders, can be particularly sensitive to their environment. Sensory overload - too much noise, too bright a light, a sudden change in their routine - can trigger a crisis. Similarly, a child who is unable to express his or her needs, or who is experiencing intense frustration, may react aggressively or shut down. The caregiver must therefore be alert to these triggers and, where possible, anticipate risky situations to prevent a crisis from escalating. For example, if they know that a child has difficulty tolerating noisy environments, they can minimize disruptive stimuli or take the child to a quiet space before the crisis escalates.

When a crisis occurs, **the caregiver's attitude is crucial**. When faced with a child in crisis, the first reaction must be to remain calm and adopt a reassuring posture. Children, especially those who don't communicate verbally or who have difficulty managing their emotions, are extremely sensitive to the emotional state of those around them. If the caregiver reacts with panic or nervousness, this is likely to aggravate the situation. On the other hand, a calm, controlled attitude can have an immediate calming effect. For example, speaking to the child in a gentle voice, using slow, predictable gestures, or simply sitting next to him without trying to touch him right away, helps the child feel safe and that the situation is under control.

**Communication** is another fundamental element in calming a child in crisis, even if the child is non-communicative or has difficulty understanding. The caregiver must adapt his or her way of communicating to the child's abilities. For a child who understands verbal language, it's important to speak slowly and explain what's going on: "I know you're angry, but it's okay, I'm here with you." This type of verbalization helps to recognize the child's emotions and make him/her understand that the caregiver is there to support him/her. If the child doesn't understand the words, the caregiver can use simple visual or tactile signals to convey the same message. Gestures such as holding out a hand, pointing to a familiar object or gently touching where the child feels safe (such as the shoulder or hand) are non-verbal ways of soothing the child.

**Adjusting the environment** is often necessary to calm a seizure. Depending on the child, it may be useful to reduce surrounding stimuli: dim the lights, turn off loud sounds or remove disturbing objects. Some children with disabilities, particularly those with autism spectrum disorders, are highly sensitive to sensory overload and need to be in a calm, predictable space to regain their emotional equilibrium. It can also be beneficial to create a comforting environment by introducing familiar objects, such as a comforter, blanket or favorite toy, which reassure the child and provide a sense of security.

Sometimes the crisis takes the form of aggressive or self-aggressive behavior, which can make it difficult to soothe the child immediately. In this case, it's essential to **reassure the child** while offering him/her space to express his/her emotions. For example, if the child starts hitting or kicking himself, it's important not to restrain him abruptly, as this could increase his frustration. Instead, the caregiver can offer alternatives to divert this negative energy, such as giving him a cushion or stress ball on which he can channel his anger in a less destructive way. It's also crucial to respect the child's personal space. Some children, especially those with cognitive difficulties, may need time alone to calm down. The caregiver must respect this need, while keeping a discreet eye on the child to make sure he or she doesn't hurt himself or put anyone else in danger.

**Soothing touch** is another technique that can be very effective in calming a child in crisis. Many children, even if they don't communicate verbally, respond positively to gentle, reassuring physical contact. This can be as simple as placing a hand gently on their back or stroking their hand. This physical contact, though seemingly minimal, can have a profound effect on a child's sense of security. For some children, particularly those with sensory difficulties, this contact can help to regulate their emotional state and reduce the intensity of the crisis. However, it's important to always respect the child's touch preferences: some children may not appreciate being touched during a seizure, and in this case, other means of soothing must be found.

Once the crisis has been defused, it is important to take the time to **soothe the child emotionally**. Once calm has returned, the caregiver can offer comfort, either through gentle words or through a moment of relaxation, such as listening to soothing music, reading a book or simply staying in a quiet environment. These post-crisis moments are essential if the child is to regain confidence and gradually understand that he or she is surrounded and supported, even when experiencing moments of great agitation or anxiety.

**Crisis prevention** is another key aspect of managing these moments. By knowing the child's potential triggers and creating a stable, predictable environment, the caregiver can anticipate certain crisis situations. This involves structuring the child's day with clear routines, avoiding abrupt changes and maintaining a sensory environment that is adapted to the child. In addition, working in collaboration with parents and the multidisciplinary team enables valuable information to be shared on the most effective strategies for preventing or managing crises.

# 4.

# Communication with children and their families

- **Understanding communication difficulties in disabled children**

Understanding communication difficulties in children with disabilities is an essential step in providing appropriate care and enabling them to express their needs, emotions and feelings. Communication, a fundamental link between the child and those around him, can be impaired by different types of disability, whether physical, sensory or cognitive. These difficulties vary widely from one child to the next, depending on the nature and severity of his or her disability, but all require special attention from healthcare professionals, and in particular care assistants. By adapting their approach and using alternative means of communication, caregivers can help the child overcome these obstacles and actively participate in his or her own care.

One of the primary sources of communication difficulties for children with disabilities is **motor disorders** affecting the muscles involved in speech. For example, a child with cerebral palsy may have muscle weakness in the mouth, tongue or throat, making it difficult or impossible to articulate words. In these cases, the child can understand what is being said, but is unable to respond verbally. These children, despite having clear ideas and desires, may find themselves locked in a forced silence, unable to share what they're feeling. This can lead to frustration, not only for the child, but also for parents and carers. It is therefore crucial to find other ways of enabling the child to express himself, by offering alternatives adapted to his physical abilities.

**Sensory disorders**, particularly hearing and visual impairments, are also a major cause of communication difficulties. A deaf or hard-of-hearing child, for example, may have difficulty understanding instructions or conversations, especially if speech is the main form of communication used around him/her. The challenge here is to find visual or gestural ways of compensating for this hearing loss. Sign language, pictograms or even electronic tablets with visual symbols can become essential tools for establishing effective communication with the child. It is important for the caregiver to learn how to use these tools and integrate them into daily care, to enable the child to understand what is going on around him/her and to participate in interactions.

**Cognitive disorders** or **developmental delays**, such as those found in children with Down's syndrome, autism or language disorders, are another source of communication difficulties. These children may have difficulty understanding verbal language, organizing their thoughts or structuring their sentences. Some autistic children, for example, may be non-verbal or use very limited language, while others may speak, but have difficulty understanding abstract concepts or following a conversation. For these children, communication becomes a more complex process, where words are not always enough to express what they feel. It is therefore necessary to adopt a simplified, structured approach to communicating with them. For example, by using short, concrete sentences, accompanying words with gestures or pictograms, and giving the child enough time to process the information and respond.

In the case of **autism spectrum disorders**, communication difficulties are not limited to verbal expression. Many autistic children also have difficulty understanding non-verbal cues, such as facial expressions, gestures or tone of voice. They may not know how to interpret other people's emotions or how to use eye contact appropriately. This can make social interactions complicated, as they don't always perceive the expectations or intentions of their interlocutors. For these children, caregivers need to adapt their body language, avoiding overly rapid gestures or complex facial expressions, and favoring clear, predictable exchanges.

**Emotional difficulties** can also interfere with communication in children with disabilities. A child who lives with constant frustration due to his inability to express his needs or make himself understood may develop aggressive behaviors, close in on himself or express his distress through tantrums. These behaviors are often an attempt to communicate an emotion or an unmet need. The caregiver must be able to recognize these behaviors as a form of communication, and seek to understand what triggers them. For example, a child may get angry because he's hungry, but can't say so clearly. In such cases, it's essential to know how to interpret these signals and respond appropriately to appease the child and meet his or her needs.

Faced with these multiple obstacles, one of the keys to improving communication with a disabled child is **the use of alternative and augmentative communication systems**. These tools can include pictograms, communication boards, touch tablets with adapted applications, or synthesized voice devices. These methods enable children to choose images or symbols to express their needs, desires or emotions. For example, a child might point to a picture of a glass of water to indicate thirst, or show a picture of a bed to indicate tiredness. These tools give children autonomy in their communication and enable them to participate actively in their care, while reducing the frustration associated with their inability to speak.

In addition to these devices, **the communication environment** must also be adapted. The caregiver needs to create a soothing environment, where the child feels comfortable expressing him/herself without pressure. This may mean slowing down the pace of interactions, giving the child time to think and respond, and avoiding overly complex or abstract questions. A child with a disability often needs extra time to process information and formulate a response. Respecting this time and not rushing them is a mark of respect and patience, which helps to build a relationship of trust.

Finally, **the relationship of trust between the child and the caregiver** is fundamental to overcoming communication difficulties. When a child feels listened to, understood and respected, he or she is more likely to open up and try to communicate, even with limited resources. The caregiver's benevolent attitude, active listening and adaptability can encourage the child to explore his or her communication skills and feel secure in expressing his or her needs.

- **Communication tools and techniques: Makaton, pictograms, etc.**

Communication tools and techniques, such as Makaton, pictograms and other alternative systems, play a crucial role in supporting children with disabilities, especially those who have difficulty expressing themselves verbally. These tools make it possible to overcome communication barriers by offering the child visual, gestural or symbolic means of sharing his or her needs, emotions and desires. They do not replace speech, but enrich or replace it when necessary, while facilitating more fluid and autonomous interaction with those around them. For caregivers, mastering these techniques is essential for establishing a relationship of trust and understanding with the child, and their regular use can greatly improve the child's quality of life by enabling him or her to be better understood.

**Makaton**, one of the most widely used methods, combines sign language and visual symbols to help children with communication difficulties express their needs and ideas. This system is particularly effective as it combines both gestures and images with words, reinforcing the child's understanding through multiple communication channels. Makaton is used not only for non-verbal children, but also for those with delayed language development or learning disabilities. Signs and symbols can be used simultaneously with speech, enabling the child to see the word, hear its pronunciation and understand its meaning through gesture. For example, to ask for "eat", the adult can show a picture of a food while making the corresponding sign with the hands and saying the word aloud. This system enriches language learning while offering children alternatives when they are unable to speak.

Makaton also has the advantage of being evolutionary. Children can start by learning a few simple signs to express basic needs such as "eating", "sleeping" or "playing", then gradually expand their vocabulary as they become more comfortable. This gradual approach enables children to learn signs at their own pace, while reinforcing their autonomy in everyday communication. The use of Makaton in a care setting is particularly valuable, as it reduces the frustration associated with the child's inability to express himself verbally, and promotes better understanding between the child, caregivers and family.

**Pictograms** are another highly effective communication tool, especially for children with cognitive difficulties or autism spectrum disorders. Pictograms are simple, clear graphic representations that enable children to understand and organize concepts or actions visually. They are often used in communication boards or visual notebooks, where the child can point to or show a pictogram to express a specific need or desire. For example, a thirsty child may point to a picture of a glass of water to indicate that he wants a drink, or use a pictogram of a toilet to indicate that he needs to go.

Pictograms are particularly useful for structuring a child's day and providing visual cues as to what's going to happen next. Pictogram-based **routine charts** are widely used to give the child a clear overview of planned activities, whether at school, at home or in a care center. Each activity is associated with a pictogram, enabling the child to anticipate and better understand the sequence of events. This visual structuring helps reduce anxiety, especially in children who have difficulty understanding unexpected changes or following complex verbal instructions. For example, a chalkboard can display images of breakfast time, playtime, tooth-brushing, or rest time, and the child can follow these steps with greater autonomy by referring to the images.

Pictograms can also be used to teach abstract or emotional concepts. For example, for a child who has difficulty identifying and expressing his emotions, a set of pictograms depicting smiling, sad, angry or frightened faces can help him better understand how he feels, and communicate these emotions to others. This becomes a valuable way of giving children an accessible emotional vocabulary, especially if they can't verbalize their feelings.

**Digital tablets and augmented communication applications**, which are becoming increasingly common, are also highly effective tools. These technologies offer an interactive platform that enables children to select images, pictograms or words to form simple sentences. Applications such as *Proloquo2Go* or *Gridper allow* children to select images representing objects, actions or emotions, then combine them to express a sentence. These systems are particularly useful for non-verbal children or those with motor difficulties, as they enable the interface to be adapted to the specific needs of each child (pictogram size, selection mode, etc.).

Tablets also offer unrivalled flexibility: they can be customized for each child according to his or her preferences and needs, and evolve as the child progresses. For example, a child may start by using simple images representing everyday objects, such as "glass", "shoes" or "bed", and over time move on to more complex concepts such as "tired", "happy" or "help me". Digital systems can also make communication more fluid and natural by offering text-to-speech, giving the child a "voice" to express himself, even if he can't speak himself.

**Natural gestures** are another alternative form of communication often used with non-verbal children or those with language difficulties. They involve the use of simple, intuitive gestures, such as pointing, waving to say hello, or raising a hand to ask for something. These gestures, although often considered basic, can be of great help to children who have not yet acquired speech, or who have difficulty organizing their thoughts verbally. Natural gestures make communication more direct and comprehensible, and are often used to complement other communication systems, such as Makaton or pictograms.

Finally, it's essential to stress that the use of these communication tools and techniques doesn't just rely on the child, but also involves **training the adults** around him - caregivers, teachers, parents. It is important that all those who interact with the child use these methods on a regular basis, so that the child can develop consistent competence in his or her communication. This requires collective learning and coordinated efforts, so that the child feels supported and encouraged to use these tools in the various contexts of his daily life.

- **Including the family in the care process: the importance of partnership**

Including the family in the care of a disabled child is fundamental to ensuring comprehensive, coherent and personalized care. The family plays a central role in the child's life, being not only his or her primary emotional support, but also a valuable source of knowledge about his or her specific needs, habits and preferences. As full partners of healthcare professionals, parents and relatives are indispensable players in supporting the child, both medically and in daily life. This partnership helps to create a harmonious and appropriate care environment, where the child feels surrounded and understood by both family and caregivers.

The importance of including the family in the care process is based first and foremost on the fact that **parents know their child intimately**. They are often the first to perceive subtle signals that caregivers don't always see. They know, for example, what soothes the child in times of anxiety, what gestures he uses to express pain, or how he prefers to be touched or approached. This parental expertise is invaluable to caregivers, who can use it to fine-tune their care. By soliciting parents' opinions, caregivers can enrich their approach, whether to better manage a crisis, choose the best communication technique, or adapt the care environment to the child's preferences.

**Communication between caregivers and families is at the heart of this partnership**. It's essential that parents feel listened to and taken into consideration in decisions concerning their child's health. Caregivers must take the time to explain each stage of care, inform parents about upcoming treatments or interventions, and answer all their questions in a transparent manner. Open communication helps to dispel fears, clarify doubts and build trust between families and healthcare professionals. For example, if a child is to undergo a particular medical treatment or rehabilitation program, caregivers must not only explain the process in understandable terms, but also listen to parents' concerns and include them in discussions about adapting the treatment to the child's reactions.

This partnership is also based on **mutual recognition of skills**. Caregivers contribute their medical expertise and professional skills, while parents bring their intimate knowledge of their child. This complementarity is crucial to providing holistic care for the child. For example, a parent may report that their child reacts badly to certain medications, or has a food intolerance that has not yet been diagnosed. Such details can guide caregivers towards therapeutic adjustments that will improve the child's quality of life. Similarly, caregivers can offer practical advice to parents on managing care at home, such as handling medical equipment or setting up appropriate hygiene routines. By working together, family and caregivers create a coherent framework for care, both in hospital and at home.

**Involving the family in daily care** also creates continuity between the child's different environments. What happens in the hospital or care center should not be disconnected from the child's daily life at home. When parents are included in the care process, they can not only better understand their child's specific needs, but also reproduce certain gestures or practices at home. For example, if a child requires regular physical therapy, parents can be trained to continue certain exercises at home, taking care not to interrupt the rehabilitation process. This continuity is essential for the well-being of the child, who should not experience a break in his or her care, and for the parents, who thus become actors in their child's daily well-being and development.

**The emotional support** the family provides for the child is another fundamental aspect of the partnership. For a child with a disability, the presence of parents or close relatives at times of care provides an emotional security that promotes the child's well-being. Medical care can be stressful, painful or disturbing for the child, and the presence of a parent by his or her side can allay fears. By their very presence, or by a comforting gesture, parents help to reduce the child's anxiety and make the experience of care more bearable. This is particularly true during invasive medical procedures or prolonged periods of hospitalization. The family then becomes a pillar of emotional support, essential if the child is to feel surrounded and secure.

Partnership with the family also enables **cultural and family preferences to be taken into account** when caring for the child. Each family has its own beliefs, values and cultural practices, which influence the way it perceives disability, illness and medical care. Including the family in the care process allows these particularities to be respected and integrated into the care plan. For example, some families may have specific dietary preferences, or particular rituals linked to care or healing. By respecting these choices and working with the family to integrate them into care, caregivers help to create a care environment that respects and values the culture and beliefs of the child and his or her loved ones.

It's also important to stress that **the family, too, needs support**. Caring for a disabled child can be emotionally and physically draining for parents, who often have to juggle home care, medical appointments, and their own professional and personal responsibilities. By including the family in the care process, caregivers can offer supportive resources, such as psychological counseling, discussion groups, or respite programs, to help parents cope with the emotional and practical burden of their child's disability. By supporting parents, caregivers indirectly contribute to the child's well-being, as supported and rested parents are better able to care for their child.

- **Managing emotions and misunderstandings: patience and pedagogy**

Dealing with the emotions and misunderstandings of a disabled child is a fundamental aspect of the caregiver's work, requiring patience and pedagogy. Children with disabilities, especially those with communication difficulties, can experience frustration, anxiety or anger when they fail to express their needs or understand what is happening to them. These emotions, often exacerbated by the disability, can manifest themselves in the form of outbursts, agitation or, on the contrary, withdrawal. Faced with these reactions, the caregiver must be able to welcome the child's emotions with kindness, while showing pedagogy to help him/her through these difficult moments.

**Patience** is the first quality needed to deal with these situations. It's important to understand that children do not experience their emotions in the same way as adults or children without disabilities. Their inability to verbalize or fully understand what's going on around them can make their reactions more intense. For example, an autistic child may be overwhelmed by an over-stimulating environment, while a child with an intellectual disability may not understand why he or she has to undergo a painful or unpleasant medical procedure. In the face of such misunderstandings, patience allows us to take the time needed to calm the child, without rushing him or imposing quick answers. This patience is expressed by slowing down the pace of care, taking a gentle approach, and repeating explanations or gestures if necessary.

The emotions of disabled children, whether anger, sadness or fear, must be **recognized and legitimized**. It is essential that the caregiver does not minimize or ignore these emotions, but instead gives them all the attention they deserve. When a child experiences an emotional crisis, the first reaction is often physical: crying, agitation, screaming. The caregiver must then take a moment to reassure the child that he or she is being heard. This may involve a simple gesture of reassurance, such as holding the child's hand or speaking softly to let him know he is safe. The caregiver's active listening is essential at these moments, as it enables the child to feel that his emotions are being taken into account, even if he can't always explain them.

**Pedagogy** is the other key to dealing with children's misunderstandings. Children with disabilities often don't immediately grasp the reasons behind certain care or activities. So it's crucial to explain what's going on, why it's necessary and what's expected of them. To do this, it's essential to use simple, clear language that's adapted to the child's ability to understand. Words must be chosen with care, and the use of visual aids, such as pictograms or images, can be a great help in illustrating explanations. For example, before taking a blood sample, the caregiver can explain to the child, using drawings or gestures, what's going to happen: "I'm going to prick you here, it's going to hurt a little, but then it'll be over." These explanations enable the child to better anticipate what he or she is going to experience, and thus reduce anxiety.

It's also important to **break tasks down into simple, accessible steps**. Faced with a situation they don't understand, children can quickly feel overwhelmed, which intensifies their anxiety. The caregiver must therefore ensure that each care or activity is presented in a fragmented way, with precise, concrete instructions, so that the child can assimilate them more easily. For example, when toileting, it's possible to say: "First we wash our hands, then we brush our teeth", accompanying these explanations with actions or visual demonstrations. This gradual, structured approach enables the child to follow instructions more serenely and accept care, even if he or she doesn't fully understand them.

**It**'s also important to **respect the child's rhythm**. Some children may need more time to process information, understand explanations or accept a new situation. In such cases, the caregiver needs to adjust his or her approach, being attentive to the child's signals, whether they be signs of discomfort, agitation or, on the contrary, withdrawal. At such moments, it is often useful to take breaks, to let the child catch his breath, and not to force the pace of care. Respecting the child's rhythm is a testament not only to the caregiver's patience, but also to his or her ability to adapt to each child's individual needs.

**Emotional support for parents** is also essential. Parents, like children, can be overwhelmed by strong emotions when they fail to understand their child's reactions or calm a crisis. The caregiver must be there to reassure and support them, explaining what is happening and giving them tools to better manage these situations. For example, he or she can show them breathing techniques or soothing gestures that they can use themselves with their child. This partnership with parents helps to create a harmonious care environment, where the child feels supported in a coherent way, both by his family and by the professionals around him.

Finally, **managing emotions and misunderstandings in children with disabilities requires constant flexibility**. Every child is different, and what works for one may not work for another. Some children may respond positively to verbal explanations, while others will need more physical reassurance or distraction to get through a difficult situation. The caregiver needs to be able to juggle these different approaches, trying out several methods until he or she finds the one that works best for each child. This ability to adjust one's approach, to observe and react according to the child's needs, is a sign of true competence and professionalism.

# 5.

# Psychological aspects of caring for disabled children

- **Recognizing and understanding children's emotional needs**

Recognizing and understanding the emotional needs of children with disabilities is fundamental to providing them with quality support that goes beyond mere physical care. A child's emotional needs, like those of an adult, are complex and influenced by many factors: his or her environment, abilities, social and family relationships, and personal experiences. For children with disabilities, these needs may be exacerbated by frustrations linked to their limitations or their difficulty in expressing what they feel. Understanding these needs, often expressed indirectly or non-verbally, is essential for healthcare professionals, and in particular for caregivers, who play a central role in the child's emotional well-being.

The first step in recognizing a child's emotional needs is to **carefully observe his or her behavior**. Children, especially those who have difficulty verbalizing their emotions, often express their emotional needs through bodily behaviors or changes in attitude. For example, a child who withdraws, avoids eye contact or refuses to participate in activities may be expressing a need for comfort or security. Conversely, a child who is agitated, cries frequently or shows signs of irritability may be expressing frustration or anxiety. The caregiver, through careful observation, must learn to decode these signals, which are not always immediately obvious, but often reflect an emotional malaise.

**The child's relational context** is also a key factor in understanding his or her emotional needs. Children with disabilities live in a context that can be both supportive and stressful. His interactions with his family, caregivers, teachers and even other children can influence his emotional state. For example, a child who lives in a highly protective family environment may have unmet needs for autonomy, while a child who feels isolated or misunderstood by his peers may express a need for attention and recognition. By taking an interest in the child's relationships with those around him, the caregiver can better understand what he's missing emotionally, and adapt the way he supports him.

It's also important to recognize that **children's emotional needs vary according to their development and disability**. Children with cognitive or intellectual disabilities may have difficulty understanding and managing their emotions. They may experience frustration when they fail to complete a task or make themselves understood, and this frustration may manifest itself in tantrums or withdrawal. These children often need increased emotional support, a reassuring presence and constant reassurance. For example, the caregiver can help them identify their emotions by verbalizing them for them: "I can see you're angry because it's hard for you to do this. It's normal, we'll work it out together." This approach helps children feel understood and supported, even if they can't always express what they're feeling.

Children with autism spectrum disorders, meanwhile, may have special emotional needs linked to heightened sensitivity to sensory stimuli. They may quickly feel overwhelmed by noisy environments, bright lights or unexpected physical contact. In this case, one of the fundamental emotional needs is to **feel safe and protected** in a calm, predictable environment. The caregiver must therefore be attentive to these sensitivities and create a soothing environment, while offering the child moments of respite when needed. For example, if a child starts to become agitated in a noisy environment, the caregiver can take him to a quieter place, reduce stimuli and give him time to refocus. This type of support, based on recognition of the child's sensory needs, is essential to enable him or her to feel emotionally secure.

**The need for comfort and affection** is another fundamental emotional need for all children, but particularly for those living with a disability. Disability can be a source of frustration, pain or a sense of difference, and children often need reassurance that they are loved and accepted as they are. The caregiver can respond to this need by offering simple but meaningful gestures, such as a smile, a gentle touch or comforting words. These gestures, however small they may seem, can have a profound impact on the child's emotional well-being. Knowing that he is surrounded by caring people who care about him and recognize his efforts helps to boost his self-esteem and ease his anxieties.

Moreover, **the need for autonomy** is often a neglected emotional need in children with disabilities. Even though they are dependent on adults for many aspects of their daily lives, these children, like all others, feel the need to make choices, take decisions and actively participate in their own lives. By respecting and encouraging this autonomy, the caregiver can help meet this essential emotional need. This can take the form of simple gestures, such as letting the child choose his or her own clothes, giving the child time to complete a task on his or her own, or encouraging the child to express his or her preferences, even if these are limited by his or her abilities. By fostering the child's autonomy, the caregiver enables him or her to feel more confident, more capable, and therefore more emotionally fulfilled.

**Managing transitions and changes** is also a crucial aspect of understanding a child's emotional needs. Children with disabilities, especially those with cognitive or sensory impairments, can be very sensitive to changes in routine or environment. An abrupt change, such as a new school, a new caregiver, or even a change in daily schedules, can generate anxiety or stress. It's therefore important to accompany these transitions gently, taking the time to explain to the child what's going to happen, using visual aids if necessary, and giving him or her time to adapt to these new situations. By being attentive to these moments of transition, the caregiver can prevent much of the emotional stress that the child may feel, and help him or her to get through these stages with greater serenity.

Finally, it's essential to **consider the family** as a resource for understanding a child's emotional needs. Parents, who know their child better than anyone else, are often the first to notice signs of emotional distress or to know what can comfort their child. Working in partnership with the family enables the caregiver to better identify the child's emotional needs and adopt a more personalized approach. What's more, the coherence between home and in-patient care promotes a stable emotional environment for the child, who feels harmoniously supported by all those around him or her.

- **Accompanying the child through difficult times: hospitalizations, operations, etc.**

Accompanying a disabled child through difficult times, such as hospitalizations or medical interventions, is a delicate and essential mission for caregivers and healthcare professionals. These situations are often a source of stress, fear and uncertainty for the child, who may feel vulnerable in the face of the medical environment and procedures he or she does not always understand. Support at these moments must be marked by kindness, patience and pedagogy, to help the child get through these ordeals as serenely as possible. The aim is not only to manage the medical aspect, but also to take care of the child's emotional well-being, offering reassuring support tailored to his specific needs.

For children with disabilities, **hospitalization** is often an upsetting experience. Children, in general, can be intimidated by the atmosphere of a hospital, with its unusual noises, bright lights, and multiple strangers in white coats. For a child with a disability, this anxiety can be exacerbated by difficulties in communication, comprehension or heightened sensitivity to sensory stimuli. Faced with this reality, the caregiver plays a key role in **establishing a climate of trust and security right from the start of hospitalization**. This involves some simple but essential gestures: introducing yourself to the child in a gentle, reassuring way, explaining what's going to happen in simple terms, and allowing the child to gradually get used to his or her new environment.

One of the first steps in accompanying a child **through** hospitalization is to **prepare the child and his or her family for this new experience**. Psychological preparation is essential to reduce anxiety. If the child is capable of understanding, it's important to explain in advance what he or she is going to experience, using appropriate aids such as drawings, pictograms or even simplified explanatory videos. These tools help to make the unknown more concrete and less frightening. For example, before a child is admitted to hospital for surgery, the caregiver can explain that he or she will meet "special doctors" who will take care of him or her, that some machines will make noises, but that he or she will be safe throughout the experience. By preparing the child in advance, the caregiver enables him or her to approach hospitalization with less fear and more understanding.

During **medical procedures,** whether invasive care or diagnostic tests, it is vital to accompany the child. These moments can be particularly stressful, as they often involve medical procedures that can be painful or impressive for the child. It is essential not to minimize the child's fear of these procedures. On the contrary, the caregiver must **recognize this fear and accompany it with empathy**. For example, he or she can hold the child's hand, talk to him or her gently to explain each step of the procedure, and remind him or her that he or she is not alone at this difficult time. Using distraction can also be an effective strategy for diverting the child's attention: a picture book, a toy or even a tablet with a cartoon can help focus the child's attention away from the procedure itself.

**Appropriate explanations of care** are also crucial during procedures. A child who doesn't understand why a blood test is necessary, or what anesthesia means, can feel very anxious. It's important to explain each step in simple, accessible terms. For example, instead of saying, "We're going to give you an injection," the caregiver can say, "You'll feel a little pinch, but it won't last long, and it'll help you feel better." Similarly, it's essential to prepare the child for the sensations he or she will experience: "You're going to have a mask over your face to help you sleep, and when you wake up, it'll all be over." This transparency and anticipation helps reduce the child's anxiety and gives him a sense of control over the situation.

**Emotional support** also plays a central role in supporting children who are hospitalized or undergoing medical procedures. The emotions these children experience, whether they be fear, sadness or frustration, must be acknowledged and handled with kindness. Children, especially those who find it difficult to verbalize their emotions, may express their stress through behaviors such as agitation, crying or withdrawal. The caregiver must be able to recognize these signals and offer appropriate support. This can take the form of gentle gestures, such as a cuddle, a hand on the shoulder, or even simply being present and listening to the child, without judging or rushing.

**The role of the family** in these moments is also essential. Parents, often just as stressed as the child, need to be involved in the care process. The caregiver must take care to reassure them and include them in every stage of care, explaining what is happening and helping them to accompany their child effectively. For example, they can show them how to reassure the child at critical moments, giving them advice on the words to use or the gestures that soothe. Family support is an invaluable resource for the child, as the presence of loved ones in difficult times provides a sense of emotional security that can alleviate the anxiety associated with hospitalization or surgery. By working closely with parents, caregivers help to strengthen the family bond and create continuity of care, from hospital to home.

In some cases, children may need **more specific stress management techniques**, such as breathing exercises or relaxation methods adapted to their age and level of understanding. These techniques can be particularly useful before a medical procedure or during waiting periods in hospital. The caregiver can teach the child simple exercises, such as breathing deeply on the count of three, or visualizing a calm, pleasant place, to help them relax. These small but simple strategies can have a significant impact on the child's hospital experience.

Finally, **post-procedure follow-up** is a key moment in the child's care. Once the operation is over, the caregiver must ensure that the child recovers in the best possible conditions, both physically and emotionally. It is important to take the time to reassure the child about what has happened, and to encourage him/her to express his/her feelings. Children can sometimes be confused or worried after a procedure, especially if they don't understand exactly what has happened to them. By explaining in simple terms that the procedure is over and that everything went well, the caregiver can help the child to regain his or her composure and feel safe.

• **Supporting parents: listening without judging**

Supporting the parents of children with disabilities is a crucial dimension of the care process. These parents, often faced with emotional, physical and organizational challenges, need caring support, listening and understanding. Listening to parents in a non-judgmental way, taking into account their difficulties and emotions, is essential to enable them to get through difficult times, manage day-to-day life better and feel less alone in their role as their child's main support. The caregiver plays a fundamental role in this support, offering a safe space where parents can express their concerns, share their emotions and find answers to their questions.

Above all, **listening without judgment** means welcoming parents into their reality, as it is, without seeking to minimize their emotions or impose solutions. Parents of disabled children often experience a range of complex emotions - from sadness and guilt to anger and helplessness. These emotions can be reinforced by the stresses of everyday life: medical appointments, regular care, the child's tantrums or uncertainty about the future. The caregiver must be able to **recognize and validate these emotions** without judging them, allowing them to be expressed freely. Sometimes, a parent may simply need to cry or express frustration without looking for immediate solutions. Being a good listener means being able to offer that space where speech is free, where there are no expectations or judgments.

The caregiver must also take into account the **emotional and physical fatigue** that parents may feel. Caring for a disabled child can be extremely exhausting, requiring constant attention, rigorous planning and management of the unexpected. Some parents may feel overwhelmed or even guilty for not doing enough, or on the contrary for doing too much and forgetting themselves. They can also be overwhelmed by a sense of isolation, especially if those around them don't fully understand the reality of their situation. At such times, it's important for the caregiver to show **compassion**, emphasizing that their feelings are legitimate and that it's normal to feel tired or overwhelmed. Simply telling a parent "You're already doing a lot, and it's normal to feel tired" may be enough to ease some of this emotional burden.

Listening without judgment also means **accepting the diversity of parental reactions** to their child's disability. Every parent reacts differently to this reality. Some immerse themselves in proactive care, seeking solutions and alternative therapies, while others may be more reticent or in denial, particularly when faced with complex situations or a difficult diagnosis. The caregiver needs to understand that every journey is unique, and that there is no "right" or "wrong" way to deal with these emotions. Some parents may be angry, others may be particularly protective or anxious, while still others will need more time to come to terms with the situation. In all cases, the caregiver must **adapt his or her approach** to the parents' personalities and needs, without ever imposing a particular path or way of reacting.

One of the fundamental aspects of supporting parents is also to **inform them in a clear and accessible way**. Faced with complex medical situations, it's easy for parents to feel lost in medical terminology, different treatments or administrative procedures. The caregiver must therefore be a point of reference, able to answer parents' questions patiently, taking the time to explain the procedures, care or options available. This clear, precise information helps to reduce parents' anxiety, as they often feel helpless in the face of uncertainty. For example, simply explaining how a procedure will be carried out, or what a particular treatment means, allows parents to better apprehend the situation and feel more involved in the care process.

In addition to listening attentively, the caregiver must **offer practical support resources** to parents. This may involve referral to associations for parents of children with disabilities, discussion groups, or respite services that give parents a break and a chance to take care of themselves. Parents are sometimes unaware of the resources available to help them cope with their daily lives. The caregiver's role is to guide them towards these solutions and encourage them to use them, without this being perceived as a sign of weakness or failure. It is essential that parents understand that they are not alone, and that asking for help or advice is not an admission of helplessness, but on the contrary, a sign of resilience and responsibility.

Finally, it is important for the caregiver **to respect the privacy and choices of the parents**. Each family has its own values, beliefs and ways of dealing with difficult situations. For example, some parents may have cultural or religious practices that influence the way they view their child's disability and care. Others may have specific expectations in terms of education or personal development. The caregiver must be able to adapt his or her support to these particularities, respecting parental choices while offering professional guidance. Respecting the diversity of families is a way of building trust between parents and caregivers, while creating a more harmonious care environment.

# 6.

# Ethics and rights for children with disabilities

- **Respecting the dignity and rights of disabled children**

Respecting the dignity and rights of children with disabilities is a fundamental principle that must guide all actions and care provided by healthcare professionals. This respect is not limited to recognizing the child's physical and medical needs; it encompasses a holistic approach that takes into account his or her emotional and psychological well-being, and right to autonomy. Every child, whatever his or her abilities or limitations, is an individual in his or her own right, with inalienable rights such as respect for his or her person, choices, needs and voice. Within this framework, the caregiver plays a key role in ensuring that the child's dignity is preserved at all times, and that his or her rights are protected and promoted.

**Respecting the child's dignity** begins with an attitude of fundamental respect in all aspects of care. The disabled child must never be reduced to his handicap; he must be perceived as a person with his own desires, preferences, emotions and individuality. This approach begins with the way we address the child. Whether they are able to communicate or not, children deserve to be treated with courtesy and kindness. It's important to talk to them directly, to include them in discussions that concern them, and not just to talk to the adults present, such as their parents or other professionals. For example, instead of asking a parent, "Does your child want something to drink?", it's better to address the child himself: "Do you want something to drink?" Even if the child can't respond verbally, it's essential that he or she feels included and considered in exchanges that concern him or her.

Respect for dignity also means **taking** into account the child's **individual preferences and needs** when providing care. Every child has his or her own limitations, but also his or her own abilities, and it's important to offer them the opportunity to actively participate in their own care. This can take the form of simple choices, such as letting the child choose the color of his or her pajamas, asking if he or she prefers to eat before or after an activity, or offering to help with toileting to the best of the child's ability. These seemingly insignificant gestures help children to feel respected as individuals, and reinforce their sense of autonomy, even in situations where they are dependent on others for care.

Respecting a child's **privacy and intimacy** is another crucial aspect of preserving his or her dignity. When a child is dependent on others for personal care, such as hygiene, dressing or medical procedures, it is essential that this care is provided with the utmost respect for the child's privacy. The caregiver must always ensure that the child is covered as much as possible during care, that doors are closed, and that gestures are carried out with delicacy and discretion. It is also important to ask for the child's consent, whenever possible, before performing any intimate care, even if the child cannot verbalize a response. For example, saying "I'm going to help you wash now" before starting a treatment helps the child understand what's happening and prepares him or her mentally for the procedure. This approach, which includes the child at every stage, gives him a voice in the care process and protects his dignity.

**The right to autonomy** is another fundamental element in respecting the dignity of the disabled child. Even if the child needs assistance with many tasks, it is important to always encourage his or her autonomy to the best of his or her ability. The child must be encouraged to participate in activities that concern his or her body and daily life. This can include gestures as simple as allowing him to brush his teeth, even if he needs help to finish, or to make decisions about his hobbies or activities. Encouraging children's autonomy shows them that they are capable, that they can have control over certain aspects of their lives, and this contributes greatly to their self-esteem. Respecting children's autonomy also means not doing for them what they can do for themselves, even if it takes longer. Patience is essential if children are to be able to do things for themselves, at their own pace.

Respect for the **rights of the child** is not limited to physical autonomy, but also encompasses the right to active participation in decisions that concern him or her. Children have the right to be informed, in a language they understand, of the treatments, care and procedures they will undergo. They also have the right to ask questions and give their opinion, to the best of their ability. Even if certain decisions have to be made by adults, it's important to always include the child in the thought process and to explain, as far as possible, the reasons for the choices being made for him or her. This can take the form of simple explanations before a medical procedure: "We're going to give you an examination to see how you're feeling and how we can help you get better", or presenting alternatives adapted to his age and understanding, such as choosing between two ways of accomplishing a task. By giving children an active role in their own care, we respect their right to expression and participation, while reinforcing their sense of control and understanding.

**The fight against stigmatization** and discrimination linked to disability is also an essential component of respect for the dignity and rights of the child. Children with disabilities are often confronted with stigmatizing or discriminatory attitudes, whether in their social environment, at school or even in certain medical contexts. The carer has a duty to combat these stereotypes by treating each child as an equal, emphasizing their abilities rather than their limitations, and ensuring that the child is included in all social or educational activities wherever possible. It's important never to make assumptions about what the child can or can't do because of their disability, but rather to offer them opportunities to express themselves and show what they can do. The caregiver must also educate other adults and children who interact with the disabled child, so that they understand that disability is not a barrier to dignity or full participation in society.

- **The caregiver's role in child protection**

The caregiver's role in child protection is vital, encompassing physical safety, emotional well-being and the safeguarding of the child's fundamental rights. When it comes to caring for children, especially those with disabilities, protection goes far beyond simply preventing accidents or illness. It's about providing a safe, caring and respectful environment, where the child can develop to the full, taking into account his or her specific needs, while preserving his or her dignity and integrity. The caregiver is at the forefront of this process, in direct contact with the child on a daily basis. His or her role in child protection is multidimensional, based on attention, vigilance, prevention and respect for the child's rights.

One of the first dimensions of this role is **physical safety**. Children with disabilities can be particularly vulnerable to environmental hazards, whether due to motor, sensory or cognitive limitations. The caregiver must ensure that the environment is adapted and safe to avoid accidents. For example, they must ensure that medical devices (such as wheelchairs or orthopedic supports) are correctly installed and used, that living spaces are clear and accessible, and that the child is always positioned to avoid falls or injury. It is also essential to keep a close eye on the child, especially during care or activities involving physical movement, to prevent any risk of injury.

However, **physical protection** is not limited to the material aspect; it also includes protection against abuse, whether physical, psychological or emotional. Children with disabilities are often more vulnerable to abuse because of their dependence on adults or their difficulty in expressing what they are experiencing. The caregiver, by virtue of his or her proximity to the child, has a particular responsibility to identify signs of abuse or neglect. These may include sudden changes in behavior, unusual physical markings, or signs of fear or withdrawal. By being alert to these clues, the caregiver can play a crucial role in detecting and preventing abuse, and alerting the appropriate authorities if necessary. It is imperative to always listen to the child, respect his or her emotions, and take seriously any indication of distress, whether expressed verbally or through behavioral changes.

**Emotional and psychological protection** is another key dimension of the caregiver's role. Children, especially those with disabilities, can be sensitive to situations of stress, anxiety or misunderstanding, often linked to their handicap or environment. The caregiver must therefore provide a reassuring and stable environment, where the child feels safe and supported. This means establishing a relationship of trust, in which the child knows he or she can count on the caregiver to protect him or her, not only physically, but also emotionally. For example, during a stressful hospitalization or medical examination, the caregiver must reassure the child with gentle gestures and explanations adapted to his age and abilities, and be there to support him every step of the way. Acknowledging and legitimizing the child's emotions, whether fear, sadness or frustration, is essential to preserving his or her psychological well-being.

As part of this emotional protection, the caregiver also plays an important role in **preserving the child's self-esteem**. Children with disabilities can sometimes feel different or marginalized because of their limitations. It is essential for the caregiver to value the child's skills and efforts, rather than focusing solely on what he or she cannot do. For example, encouraging the child to take part in activities, make choices or perform tasks suited to his or her abilities helps build self-confidence. The caregiver must always adopt a positive approach, valuing the child's small successes, and offering opportunities to exercise autonomy, even in simple everyday gestures.

**Respect for children's rights** is another fundamental aspect of protection. All children, including those with disabilities, have rights that must be respected, including the right to education, expression, protection from abuse and a family life. The caregiver has a responsibility to ensure that these rights are protected, working with parents, educators and other healthcare professionals to provide an environment that respects the child's dignity and needs. For example, the caregiver must ensure that the child has the opportunity to express himself, even if he cannot do so verbally, using adapted communication tools such as pictograms or sign language. The child's right to be heard is essential, and the caregiver must ensure that the child can actively participate in his or her own care, to the best of his or her ability.

**Risk prevention** is also a central aspect of the caregiver's role in child protection. This involves anticipating risky situations and putting measures in place to avoid them. For example, if a child is particularly vulnerable to infection because of his or her state of health, the caregiver must ensure that all hygiene measures are rigorously observed, that the child is vaccinated, and that he or she is protected from unnecessary exposure to germs. In the same spirit, it is important to adapt care to the child's specific needs, taking into account any physical or cognitive limitations, to avoid any complications. Prevention also includes training and raising the awareness of other people who interact with the child, to ensure that everyone understands and complies with safety protocols.

Finally, **collaboration with the family** is a crucial aspect of child protection. The child's parents or legal guardians are often the primary protectors of his or her well-being, and the caregiver must work closely with them to ensure harmonious care. This means informing parents of all care procedures, including them in important decisions, and supporting them in their role as parents. Sometimes, it also means making them aware of certain aspects of child protection, such as the signs of abuse, the risks associated with certain practices, or the importance of fostering the child's autonomy in everyday activities. This collaboration helps to create a care environment in which the child feels protected by both family and professionals.

- **Handling delicate situations: abuse, failure to respect children's needs**

Dealing with delicate situations such as abuse or failure to respect a child's needs is a crucial responsibility for all caregivers. In the course of their work, they may be confronted with situations where children, particularly those with disabilities, are vulnerable, neglected or abused, whether intentionally or by omission. These situations demand special attention, immediate responsiveness and delicate management, as they affect the child's safety and well-being. The caregiver must not only be able to detect signs of abuse or neglect, but also know how to intervene appropriately and follow the protocols in place to protect the child while avoiding creating further trauma.

**Detecting signs of abuse or neglect** is an essential first step. Abuse can take many forms: physical, emotional, psychological, even sexual. It can also take the form of neglect, i.e. the absence of adequate care, food or security. For children with disabilities, abuse or neglect can be more difficult to identify, as they may be unable to express themselves clearly or to report the abuse. The caregiver, who is in daily contact with the child, needs to be **alert to warning signs**. These may include physical signs, such as unexplained bruises, burns or cuts, or emotional and behavioral signs, such as abrupt changes in the child's attitude, social withdrawal, abnormal fear of adults or anxiety attacks. Similarly, signs of neglect, such as poor hygiene, inappropriate clothing or chronic fatigue, may indicate that the child's basic needs are not being met.

When these signs appear, the caregiver must be **vigilant and discerning**. It's important not to jump to conclusions, but rather to take the whole context into account. For example, some behaviors or injuries may be related to features of the child's disability (such as frequent falls for a child with motor difficulties), while others may signal a more serious problem. In all cases, the caregiver must document these observations rigorously and in detail, noting dates, precise descriptions of signs and any suspicious behavior, so as to build up a clear record in the event of necessary intervention.

**Communication with the child** is essential in managing these delicate situations. When a child with a disability is potentially abused or neglected, he or she may find it difficult to express what he or she is experiencing, either because of communication limitations, fear or shame. It is therefore important for the caregiver to develop a relationship of trust with the child, where the latter feels safe enough to express his or her emotions or concerns. The caregiver needs to be patient and attentive, using appropriate communication techniques such as pictograms or simple gestures to encourage the child to share what he or she is feeling or has experienced. For example, if children are unable to verbalize their experiences, they can be invited to point to images that represent different emotions or situations. This approach allows the child to express himself without having to resort to words he doesn't master, while providing a reassuring framework for revealing important information.

**When suspicions of abuse or disregard for a child's needs arise**, the caregiver has an obligation to act quickly, while respecting current reporting protocols. In most care structures or institutions, there are clear procedures to follow in the event of suspected abuse, which include reporting to internal officials (such as a referring doctor or coordinator) or to competent external services, such as social services or child protection. The caregiver should never attempt to resolve the situation alone, or directly accuse a person without formal proof. It's crucial to respect **communication channels and legal** procedures, to ensure that the intervention is carried out correctly and that the child's safety comes first.

However, in these critical moments, it is also important to **protect the child emotionally**. The reporting or investigation process can be stressful for a child, especially if he or she is already in an abusive situation. The caregiver must ensure that the child feels supported, understood and secure during this period. They should avoid asking intrusive questions or seeking direct confessions, as this could further traumatize the child or prejudice an ongoing investigation. The caregiver's role is above all to remain an emotional anchor for the child, offering a space to listen and comfort, while taking care not to aggravate the child's distress.

**Prevention** is another essential aspect of managing delicate situations such as abuse or failure to respect a child's needs. The caregiver can play an active role in raising awareness among families, colleagues and other professionals around the child of the risks of abuse and the specific needs of children with disabilities. They can also help to **create a respectful and protective care environment**, where the child's physical, emotional and social needs are always taken into account. This involves regular training in managing difficult behavior, understanding the special needs of disabled children, and creating a caring, inclusive environment where every child feels valued and protected.

Respecting children's needs goes beyond simply preventing abuse. It means **ensuring that every child receives the care appropriate** to his or her condition, without neglect or discrimination. Some disabled children may have complex medical or psychological needs, and it is the caregiver's duty to ensure that these needs are respected. This means, for example, adapting care to the child's abilities, avoiding any form of brutality or impatience, and ensuring that the child is always treated with dignity and respect. Any form of neglect, whether intentional or unintentional, can have serious consequences for the child's development and well-being, and it is essential that the caregiver ensures that the child receives all the attention he or she needs.

- **Work in accordance with laws and regulations in the
  medical-social field**

Working in accordance with the laws and regulations of the
medico-social sector is a fundamental responsibility for all
healthcare professionals, including care assistants. In this sector,
laws and regulations are not simply abstract rules: they are
designed to guarantee the quality of care, protect the rights of
patients, especially the most vulnerable, and frame professional
practices to maintain a safe, ethical and respectful care
environment. Caregivers, as actors in the field, must understand
and respect these legal and ethical frameworks in order to
contribute to the smooth running of the care system, protect
patients and ensure that practices comply with legal requirements.

Laws and regulations in the medico-social field touch on several
aspects of care, including **patient rights**, confidentiality of
information, working conditions for caregivers, and standards of
safety and quality of care. **Patients' rights** play a central role in
these regulations. In France, for example, the March 4, 2002 law
on patients' rights and the quality of the healthcare system
established fundamental principles to protect the rights of
healthcare system users. This law enshrines the right to
information, the right to consent, and respect for privacy and
dignity. For caregivers, this means that they must inform patients
in a clear and comprehensible manner about the care they are
receiving, respect their choices and obtain their informed consent
before any intervention, even for the simplest acts of care. For
example, before providing hygiene care to a disabled child or
adult, it is essential to explain what is going to be done, and to
ensure the patient's agreement, insofar as he or she is capable of
understanding and responding.

**Confidentiality** of medical and personal information is another
pillar of regulation in the medical-social field. By virtue of
medical secrecy, care assistants are required to guarantee the
confidentiality of information relating to patients' health. This
means that any information concerning a patient's state of health,
treatment or living conditions must never be divulged to third

parties without the consent of the patient or his/her legal representatives. This obligation of confidentiality extends to all professional interactions and to written or digital media. For example, a caregiver must never discuss a patient's health information with anyone outside the care team directly concerned, and must ensure that medical records are well protected against unauthorized access. Respecting this confidentiality is not only a legal requirement, but also an essential element in maintaining trust between caregiver and patient.

In addition to patients' rights, care assistants must also ensure that **their work complies with standards of safety and quality of care**. The medical-social field is heavily regulated to ensure that the care provided complies with safety and quality standards, in order to prevent medical errors, nosocomial infections and other care-related risks. Caregivers are trained to apply these standards in their day-to-day work, by following hygiene protocols, ensuring the correct use of medical equipment, and following rigorous procedures for each treatment. For example, washing hands before and after each treatment, using gloves and disinfectants, and carefully checking medical devices before use are all daily gestures that reflect respect for these safety standards. These practices, which are enshrined in regulations, are designed to protect both patients and caregivers from care-related risks.

Caregivers must also **be familiar with laws specific to the medico-social field**, particularly those concerning the care of vulnerable people, such as children, the elderly or people with disabilities. In France, for example, the February 11, 2005 law on equal rights and opportunities, participation and citizenship for the disabled profoundly altered the legal framework for the care of the disabled. This law guarantees access to care, education and social inclusion for disabled people, and requires medical-social establishments to adapt to meet their specific needs. For a caregiver, this means ensuring that the care provided respects these principles of equality and inclusion, by ensuring that disabled people have access to the same care and rights as other patients. This may include adaptations in the way they communicate, in the organization of care or in the layout of equipment to meet the specific needs of each patient.

As part of their daily work, orderlies must also be aware of their **legal and professional responsibilities**. In France, the Public Health Code governs the practice of healthcare professionals, including orderlies. It defines the acts that orderlies are authorized to perform under the responsibility of a nurse, as well as their professional obligations. This includes requirements in terms of ongoing training, professional ethics and compliance with care protocols. Caregivers must know the limits of their competence, and know when it is necessary to call in a nurse or doctor to intervene. Failure to meet these obligations, or to comply with regulations, may result in sanctions, up to and including professional suspension or disbarment. So, caregivers must always be aware of the legal implications of their actions, and ensure that they are working in accordance with the regulations in force.

**Reporting situations of risk or abuse** is another legal obligation in the medical-social field. If a caregiver witnesses or suspects a situation of abuse, neglect or violence towards a patient, he or she is required to report it immediately to the appropriate authorities. In France, this reporting obligation is enshrined in the Penal Code and the Code de l'action sociale et des familles. Failure to report abuse may result in prosecution for failure to assist a person in danger. Caregivers must therefore be vigilant and know how to react to such situations, following legal procedures to protect the patient while respecting the rights of all those involved.

Finally, **the working conditions of** care assistants are also governed by regulations designed to guarantee their safety and well-being. Work in the medical-social sector can be physically and emotionally demanding, and it is important that caregivers work in conditions that respect their health and dignity. This includes respect for working hours, break times, protective measures against physical risks (such as musculoskeletal disorders linked to carrying heavy loads), and consideration of psychosocial risks. Occupational health regulations, such as the right to ongoing training and psychological support, are designed to protect caregivers and enable them to carry out their duties in the best possible conditions.

# 7.

# Helping disabled children get into school

- **The caregiver's role in school support**

The caregiver's role in supporting children with disabilities at school is essential to their inclusion, well-being and educational success. In a school setting, the caregiver provides essential support, ensuring that the child's specific needs are taken into account, whether physical, medical or emotional. This role goes far beyond simply assisting with daily tasks, as it also helps to promote the child's autonomy, facilitate learning and reinforce social integration. As a supportive member of the educational team, the caregiver helps to create an inclusive, secure and caring school environment, where children can flourish despite their difficulties.

**Providing daily care** is one of the caregivers' primary responsibilities in the school environment. Children with disabilities may have specific medical or physical needs that require regular assistance during the school day. This may include help with toileting, monitoring the administration of medication, or assistance with meals. For example, a child with motor difficulties may need help to move around, sit properly in class, or use technical aids such as a wheelchair. The caregiver ensures that these needs are met discreetly and respectfully, so that the child can participate fully in school life without his or her disability becoming an insurmountable obstacle. They also play a role in preventing health complications, by being alert to signs of fatigue, pain or discomfort, and intervening quickly if necessary.

In this context, the caregiver helps to **promote the child's autonomy**. It's not just a question of assisting the child in all his tasks, but of encouraging him to do what he can do by himself, respecting his rhythm and valuing his abilities. For example, a child who has difficulty dressing himself can be encouraged to try on certain items of clothing or fasten his shoes, even if he needs help to finish. This kind of progressive support is essential to boost the child's self-confidence and show him that he is capable of accomplishing things despite his limitations. The caregiver plays a guiding role here, providing the necessary assistance while fostering the development of skills that will be useful not only at school, but also in everyday life.

**Facilitating the child's participation in school activities** is another important aspect of support. Some children with disabilities may have difficulty keeping up with the pace of lessons or participating in group activities, whether due to physical limitations or cognitive difficulties. The caregiver helps to adapt these activities to the child's abilities, working closely with teachers and other school professionals. For example, if a child has difficulty writing due to reduced fine motor skills, the caregiver can help him/her to hold an adapted pencil or to use a computer with an ergonomic keyboard. Similarly, for a child with attention or concentration problems, the caregiver can help him or her to stay focused by suggesting tools such as visual cards, or by giving clear cues as to what needs to be done. This role of pedagogical support is essential if the child is not to be excluded from the learning process, and if he or she is to progress at his or her own pace, while taking an active part in classroom activities.

In addition to individual support, the caregiver plays a crucial role **in the child's social integration within the school**. The school environment can sometimes be a source of stress for a child with a disability, particularly due to interactions with peers or perceived differences. The caregiver's presence and support can help facilitate these interactions, ensuring that the child does not feel isolated or marginalized. He or she can encourage the child to take part in group games, recreational activities and collaborative projects, taking care to adapt situations so that he or she can take part. For example, if a child finds it difficult to run or take part in sports activities, the caregiver can help suggest alternatives or raise awareness among the other children so that they include their comrade in adapted games.

The caregiver can also **play a mediating** role in relations between the disabled child and his or her peers. Children can sometimes lack understanding or awareness of the particularities of their disabled peers, which can lead to misunderstandings or situations of exclusion. The caregiver can help explain the child's needs to the other pupils, using simple words and encouraging them to be caring and cooperative. For example, he or she can explain that certain tasks are more difficult for the child, but that he or she can do them with a little more time or help, and thus encourage mutual aid and respect. This social integration work is essential if children are to feel at ease in their school environment, and build positive relationships with their peers.

In addition to their day-to-day duties, caregivers must also **work closely with teachers and other** school **professionals.** This collaboration is essential to ensure that the child's needs are fully understood and taken into account in all aspects of his or her school life. The caregiver can provide valuable information on the child's specific needs, abilities and limitations, so that teachers can adapt their teaching methods accordingly. For example, he or she may inform a teacher that a child needs more frequent breaks or a quiet environment in which to concentrate, or that he or she needs more time to complete certain tasks. This constant dialogue enables us to adjust educational practices and ensure that the child benefits from an inclusive and adapted learning environment.

In addition, the caregiver can play a key role in **the orientation and follow-up of personalized educational projects** (PEP or PPS in France). These plans are put in place to define the adaptations required for the schooling of children with disabilities, according to their specific needs. The caregiver, who knows the child well, can take part in meetings to monitor these plans and contribute his or her expertise on what works best for the child in terms of support, material or educational adaptations. This contribution is invaluable in fine-tuning educational strategies and ensuring that the child receives comprehensive support that enables him or her to progress under the right conditions.

Finally, **the emotional aspect** of school support must not be overlooked. The caregiver plays a moral support role for the child, acting as a reassuring point of reference in an environment that can sometimes be a source of stress or anxiety. During difficult moments - an assessment, a complicated social interaction, or a day when the child feels more vulnerable - the caregiver is there to listen, comfort and encourage the child to persevere. This invaluable support helps children to manage their emotions and stay motivated, even in the face of the challenges of schooling.

- **Working with teachers and AVSs (auxiliaires de vie scolaire)**

Working in collaboration with teachers and Auxiliaires de Vie Scolaire (AVS) is essential to provide the best possible support for children with disabilities in the context of their schooling. This cooperation enables a comprehensive response to the child's educational, social and health needs, while promoting his or her inclusion in the school environment. The caregiver's specific role, centered on the child's care and physical well-being, makes him or her part of a multidisciplinary team whose aim is to ensure harmonious, coherent care adapted to each situation. Complementarity between these different players is the key to successful support, where each professional brings his or her own expertise to bear on the child's overall development.

**Working with teachers** is a central dimension of this collaboration. Teachers, who are on the front line of pedagogical support, have in-depth knowledge of the child's educational needs, strengths and challenges in the classroom. However, they may not always have the specific skills to meet the child's medical, physical or sensory needs. This is where the caregiver plays a crucial role. They bring their expertise to bear on the care and adaptations needed to ensure that the child can attend classes in the best possible conditions. For example, if a child needs special arrangements to sit comfortably, or regular breaks to avoid fatigue, the caregiver can inform the teacher and suggest appropriate solutions. Similarly, he or she can make the teacher aware of any medical particularities, such as when the child should take medication, or what gestures to avoid to avoid causing pain or discomfort.

This collaboration also involves **a regular exchange of information** between the caregiver and the teacher. Every day, the caregiver is in direct contact with the child, and can observe changes in his or her behavior, state of health or mood, which may influence his or her ability to follow the lessons. By communicating these observations to the teacher, the caregiver can adapt teaching methods and the organization of the school day to the child's immediate needs. For example, if the caregiver notices that the child is particularly tired or anxious, he or she can suggest that the teacher modulate certain activities or schedule rest periods. This reactivity ensures that the child remains in a supportive and caring learning environment, while respecting his or her limits.

**Auxiliaires de Vie Scolaire (AVS)** also play a vital role in supporting children with disabilities. AVSs are specifically trained to help children with their daily tasks at school, assisting them with mobility, writing, material management and social integration with other pupils. However, AVSs are not health professionals, and this is where the caregiver complements their action. This may involve, for example, providing specific care that the AVS cannot provide, or monitoring any medical complications linked to the child's state of health. Collaboration between the caregiver and the AVS is therefore essential to ensure that the child's needs are met from both an educational and a medical point of view.

A good example of this complementarity is the case of a child requiring regular care or with mobility problems. The AVS can help the child move around the school, take part in class activities and interact with classmates, while the caregiver intervenes to provide more technical care or monitor the child's health. This complementarity enables each person to remain within his or her field of expertise, while ensuring that the child benefits from comprehensive support, both medical and educational. This sharing of tasks also avoids the risk of burnout for one or other of the professionals, as each knows what falls within his or her field of intervention.

**Coordination between the caregiver, teacher and AVS** requires fluid, regular communication. Consultative meetings or informal exchanges at the beginning or end of the day are often essential to adjust the child's support according to changing needs. These moments of exchange enable us to adapt our practices, share information on the child's health or progress at school, and reflect together on strategies to improve inclusion and participation in the classroom. For example, if a child shows signs of physical improvement, the caregiver can inform the AVS and teacher that the child is now able to perform certain tasks more independently, and they can adjust the level of support accordingly. Conversely, if the child's health deteriorates, a reassessment of his or her needs may be necessary to provide a more suitable school environment.

**The emotional support** the caregiver can provide to teachers and AVSs is also an important aspect of this collaboration. Caring for children with disabilities, especially those with complex needs, can be challenging for the professionals who look after them on a daily basis. Teachers and care assistants can sometimes feel helpless or at a loss when faced with medical situations beyond their control. Thanks to their expertise and experience, caregivers can reassure their colleagues by providing clear information on the child's medical needs, and helping them to adapt their practice without fear of making mistakes. For example, he can explain to teachers how to react in the event of a medical crisis or extreme fatigue, or reassure them about the appropriate gestures to adopt during basic care, such as helping a child to sit up or stand up. This support helps to create a more serene working atmosphere, where every member of the team feels able to contribute fully to the child's care.

**Training and awareness-raising** are also important tools in this collaboration. With their knowledge of the child's specific needs and the pathologies associated with his or her disability, caregivers can act as trainers for teachers and AVSs. For example, they can teach them how to use certain medical equipment, such as a wheelchair or breathing aid, or explain how to adapt exercises to the child's physical abilities. In addition, he or she can make the entire educational team aware of the warning signs of discomfort, crisis or fatigue, so that they can react quickly and appropriately. This transmission of knowledge and know-how is essential if all those involved are to be able to work together effectively and in the child's best interests.

- **Integration of children in specialized vs. regular schools**

The integration of children with disabilities into specialized versus mainstream schools is a central issue in the field of inclusive education. Each of these two approaches presents advantages and challenges, and the choice between one or the other often depends on the child's specific needs, the nature of his or her disability, and the ability of the structures to respond adequately to these needs. The aim, whatever the setting, is always to guarantee the child a development-friendly environment, where he or she can not only receive a quality education, but also develop personally, socially and emotionally. Understanding the issues at stake in these two models enables us to better understand the benefits of inclusive education, while recognizing the importance of specialized institutions in certain cases.

**Ordinary schools** represent the model of inclusive education, where children with disabilities are integrated into mainstream classes with children without disabilities. This model aims to promote equal opportunities, social inclusion and the participation of all students, whatever their abilities or particularities. In this context, children benefit from the same education as their peers, while receiving, if necessary, support adapted to their specific needs. This support can take the form of educational adjustments, such as the adaptation of teaching methods or materials, or the presence of school life assistants (AVS) or care assistants to help the child with his or her daily needs.

One of the main **advantages of integration into a mainstream school environment** is that it fosters socialization and inclusion. By attending school alongside children without disabilities, disabled children develop rich and varied social interactions, learn to evolve in a diverse environment, and benefit from positive role models. This mix is beneficial for all children, as it helps them to better understand the diversity of individuals and to accept differences from an early age. Children with disabilities can feel fully integrated into society, rather than isolated or marginalized. What's more, being in an ordinary environment enables the child to be confronted with expectations similar to those of other pupils, which can stimulate his or her cognitive, emotional and social development.

Integration into a mainstream school can also be **academically stimulating**, as it exposes the child to diversified teaching and pedagogical practices adapted to individual skills. The child can benefit from a personalized schooling project (PPS), which defines the adjustments required to enable him/her to follow the curriculum under the right conditions. For example, a child with learning difficulties may be provided with adapted teaching aids, such as visual aids, digital tools or differentiated assessments, while a child with motor difficulties may be provided with aids to facilitate his or her physical integration into the classroom.

However, **integration into mainstream schools** also presents challenges. Not all schools have the resources needed to welcome children with disabilities in the best possible way. For example, some schools may lack adapted infrastructure (such as access ramps or elevators), or staff trained to meet the specific needs of children with disabilities. What's more, in some classes, the pace of teaching or the size of the class may make it difficult to adapt to the individual needs of each pupil, and the child with a disability may not receive the attention he or she needs. This can lead to frustration, both for the child and for teachers, who have to juggle the needs of all pupils. So, although inclusion in a mainstream school is an ideal to be achieved, it is not always possible or beneficial if the means put in place are not sufficient to guarantee the child's well-being.

**Specialized schools** are specifically designed to meet the needs of children with disabilities. They offer infrastructures, educational programs and teams of professionals adapted to each type of disability. These establishments can accommodate children with severe or complex disabilities, who require constant medical attention, specialized care or highly individualized pedagogy. Unlike ordinary schools, these establishments often have on-site medical and paramedical services, such as physiotherapists, speech therapists and psychomotor therapists, who can intervene directly as part of the school day.

**One of the great advantages of specialized schools** is their ability to offer highly personalized support, tailored to each child's abilities and needs. Class sizes are generally small, enabling teachers and other health professionals to concentrate more intensively on the care of each child. Teaching is often much more flexible, with teaching methods adapted to the cognitive, sensory or motor particularities of the pupils. For example, a visually impaired child might benefit from specific tools to learn in Braille, while a child with severe autistic disorder might be supervised by a team trained in educational methods specific to this type of disability, such as the TEACCH method or applied behavior analysis (ABA). This type of personalization, which is more difficult to implement in ordinary schools, enables the child to progress at his or her own pace and benefit from tailor-made support.

**Specialized establishments** also offer a setting where children can feel confident, surrounded by professionals who fully understand their needs. Children evolve in a structured environment, where every detail is designed to promote their well-being and development. This can be particularly reassuring for children with serious disorders or complex medical needs, who require constant supervision. For example, a child with severe epilepsy may need rapid medical attention in the event of a seizure, which is easier to manage in a facility where health professionals are permanently on hand.

However, specialized institutions are not without their challenges either. One **potential drawback** is that they can, in some cases, isolate children from their peers without disabilities, limiting their interactions with children from diverse backgrounds. This separation can sometimes create a sense of disconnection from society as a whole, or reinforce the idea that the child is "different". Although these facilities offer highly specialized services, they can sometimes miss out on opportunities to socialize with children from all backgrounds, which is a key element in a child's social and emotional development. What's more, some parents may fear that their child is not sufficiently prepared to face the reality of the outside world after having been schooled in a highly protected environment.

- **How to adapt school and teaching materials to children's needs**

Adapting school and teaching materials to the needs of children with disabilities is an essential step in promoting their inclusion and guaranteeing their access to education. Children with physical, sensory or cognitive disabilities often require specific adaptations to enable them to participate fully in school activities and benefit from quality teaching. These adaptations are not limited to tools or equipment alone, but also include adjustments to teaching methods, learning materials and classroom organization. The aim is to create an inclusive learning environment, where each child can flourish and progress according to his or her abilities, while taking an active part in the life of the class.

One of the first steps in adapting school equipment is to **take into account the** child's **type of disability**, in order to choose the most appropriate tools. For children with **motor disabilities**, adaptation often concerns equipment that facilitates their mobility and posture in the classroom. For example, a child in a wheelchair may need a height-adjustable or tilted desk to write comfortably. Supports to stabilize the arm or hand when writing can also be useful for children with fine motor disorders. In addition, for children with difficulties in manipulating objects, the use of ergonomic pencils and pens, which are easier to hold, or voice recognition software to write their work can greatly facilitate their participation in school activities.

For children with **sensory difficulties**, such as visual or hearing impairments, adaptations to the equipment must enable them to compensate for these sensory limitations and access the same information as their peers. For visually impaired or blind children, **adapted visual aids** are essential. This includes the use of Braille texts, large-print textbooks, or tablets and computers equipped with voice synthesis and screen-reading software. In addition, interactive boards or tactile devices can offer a more accessible visual alternative, with high contrasts and colors adapted to the child's needs. For deaf or hard-of-hearing children, it's crucial to install equipment such as **magnetic loop systems that** amplify sounds, or subtitles for video material, so that they can follow lessons with the same level of access as other pupils. What's more, in some cases, adaptation can include learning sign language for the child and his or her classmates, to facilitate communication within the classroom.

**Cognitive** or specific learning **disorders**, such as dyslexia, dyscalculia or attention deficit hyperactivity disorder (ADHD), also require specific adaptations to teaching materials. For dyslexic children, the use of **adapted fonts**, such as OpenDyslexic, which facilitates reading by making letters more distinct, can greatly improve reading comfort. Similarly, access to audio books or text-to-speech software enables children to bypass their reading difficulties while still accessing the content of school textbooks. For children with attention disorders, it can be useful to provide **structured visual aids**, such as planning boards or clear, prioritized task lists, to help them concentrate and organize their work more effectively. In this case, tools such as visual timers or noise-cancelling headphones can also be useful in reducing distractions and improving their concentration.

**Adapting teaching methods** is another important aspect of supporting children with disabilities. Teaching materials need to be flexible and diversified, to accommodate different learning styles. Some children learn better visually, others by touching or listening. It is therefore important to offer a variety of supports and tools, such as diagrams, videos, hands-on activities and interactive educational games, to enable each child to appropriate knowledge in the way that suits him best. For example, for a child with abstract comprehension difficulties, teachers can use **concrete manipulatives**, such as physical objects to illustrate mathematical concepts, to make learning more tangible and understandable.

The organization of the classroom itself can be adapted to facilitate access to materials and learning. It's essential to **create an inclusive and accessible classroom environment**, where every child feels comfortable and supported. This can include physical adaptations, such as arranging furniture to allow wheelchair users to move around, or providing a quiet corner for children who need temporary isolation from excessive sensory stimuli. The layout of teaching aids can also be rethought, for example by placing learning tools within easy reach of children who have difficulty moving around, or by organizing workshops in small groups to encourage interaction and mutual support.

In addition to equipment and the physical organization of the classroom, adaptation can also include the **training of teachers** and other school staff. It's crucial that teachers are trained in the specific needs of disabled children, and are familiar with the teaching tools and techniques best suited to their situation. For example, a teacher can learn to use text-to-speech software, or adapt lessons to include regular breaks for children with attention deficit disorders. What's more, it's important that the entire educational team, including AVSs and care assistants, work in a coordinated fashion to ensure that the child benefits from comprehensive, coherent support.

**Dialogue with parents** also plays an essential role in adapting school materials. Parents are often in the best position to understand their child's specific needs, and can provide valuable information on tools or techniques that work well at home. Close collaboration between parents, teachers, carers and other professionals helps to identify the adaptations needed, and to ensure that the child benefits from a coherent learning environment, both at school and at home.

Finally, it's important to stress that **adapting school equipment should not stigmatize the child**, but rather help him or her to feel integrated into the classroom and able to follow lessons like their peers. Adaptations should be designed to enhance the child's abilities and reinforce his autonomy, rather than emphasizing his difficulties. For example, instead of focusing on the child's limitations, the emphasis should be on the tools that enable him to bypass these obstacles and participate fully in school activities. In addition, it is essential that other students are made aware of the importance of inclusion, and that they understand that each child may have specific needs, without this making him or her fundamentally different from others.

- **Emotional support for learning difficulties**

Emotional support in the face of learning difficulties is a fundamental aspect of support for children, especially those with disabilities. When a child is faced with obstacles to learning, whether cognitive, behavioral or sensory, he or she may experience a multitude of emotions: frustration, discouragement, loss of self-confidence, even anxiety. If these emotions are not recognized and managed, they can exacerbate difficulties at school, leading to a vicious circle in which the child feels increasingly out of step with his or her peers. Caregivers, teachers and all other professionals involved in the child's life play an essential role in providing emotional support to help the child overcome his or her difficulties and regain confidence in his or her abilities.

One of the first steps in supporting a child with learning difficulties is to **recognize and legitimize his or her emotions**. When a child finds himself in a situation of failure or difficulty, it's crucial to make him understand that his feelings are normal and legitimate. Telling a child "I can see you're frustrated, it's normal, everyone has difficulties" validates their feelings and shows them they're not alone in their emotions. This recognition is essential if the child is not to feel misunderstood or isolated in his or her learning journey. The caregiver, often in close contact with the child, can play an important role in identifying these moments of discouragement and offering immediate emotional support, reassuring the child that his difficulties do not define him, and that they can be overcome.

**Encouraging perseverance and valuing effort** is another key component of emotional support. A child facing learning difficulties can quickly lose self-confidence, especially if he perceives his efforts as futile or if he constantly compares himself to his peers who are making faster progress. That's why it's essential to value every little bit of progress, every effort made, no matter how small. For example, if a dyslexic child manages to read a few words unaided after several attempts, it's important to celebrate this achievement and show him that his efforts are bearing fruit. The caregiver, in collaboration with the teachers, must ensure that a positive and encouraging attitude is adopted, highlighting progress rather than failure. This approach enables the child to understand that learning is a gradual process, and that he or she has the ability to progress at his or her own pace.

In some cases, learning difficulties can be a source of **intense frustration or anxiety**, particularly if the child feels overwhelmed or unable to meet expectations. This anxiety can manifest itself in avoidance behavior, agitation or, on the contrary, withdrawal. The caregiver needs to be alert to these signals and offer solutions to reduce this pressure. This can include simple relaxation techniques, such as breathing exercises to help the child manage stress, or moments of pause and relaxation to help the child refocus. **Intermediate goals** can also be set, breaking down complex tasks into smaller, more manageable steps. For example, if a child is having difficulty solving a math problem, the caregiver can suggest that he or she first concentrate on one part of the problem, then progress step by step, thus reducing anxiety about a task perceived as too difficult.

**Good communication** is also a fundamental tool for emotional support. It's important for the child to feel listened to and understood, and to be able to express his frustrations without fear of being judged. The caregiver, by virtue of his or her daily proximity to the child, can play the role of a confidant, a person of trust to whom the child can turn when feeling overwhelmed. By adopting an active listening posture, the caregiver can help the child put words to his emotions, better understand his own reactions, and feel supported in his journey. This caring dialogue helps to defuse tense situations and offers the child a safe space in which to express his fears, doubts and feelings.

**Reinforcing the child's self-esteem** is also a crucial dimension of emotional support. Children with learning difficulties can quickly develop a negative self-image, perceiving themselves as "less capable" than their peers. The caregiver, in conjunction with teachers, must counterbalance this perception by highlighting the child's talents and skills, even outside the school environment. For example, a child with reading difficulties can be encouraged in his artistic or sporting talents, or in his ability to interact positively with his peers. By emphasizing a child's strengths, we show them that their learning difficulties do not define their identity, and that they have many other skills to explore and develop.

Another important aspect of emotional support is **helping parents** to manage their child's difficulties. Parents can also be emotionally affected by their child's learning difficulties, and it's crucial to include them in the support process. The carer can act as a link between the school and the family, keeping parents informed of the child's progress, the strategies put in place to help, and offering advice on how to support their child at home. This collaborative approach helps to create a coherent framework around the child, where academic efforts are reinforced by caring and encouraging family support.

Finally, it's essential to create an **inclusive, non-competitive school environment**, where every child feels respected and supported, whatever their level of performance. The caregiver, in collaboration with teachers, can ensure that the classroom is a place where children do not feel in constant competition with their peers, but where their efforts are valued and encouraged. Setting up group activities, where each child can contribute according to his or her skills, helps to reinforce cooperation and mutual support, rather than focusing on individual performance. This collective approach reduces the pressure felt by children in difficulty, enabling them to invest in learning without fear of judgment or failure.

# 8.

# Support for leisure and social activities

- **The importance of leisure in the development of disabled children**

Leisure time plays a crucial role in the development of children with disabilities, just as it does for other children. It's not just a time to relax or have fun, but a fundamental space for learning, personal development and socialization. Leisure activities enable children to develop their physical, social, emotional and cognitive skills in a setting that is less structured than school, but just as important for their overall development. For children with disabilities, leisure can also provide specific opportunities to build their self-confidence, overcome perceived limitations, and interact with their peers in an inclusive and rewarding setting.

**Developing physical skills** is one of the first positive aspects that leisure activities can bring to children with disabilities. Physical activities such as adapted sports, swimming or outdoor games help to improve motor skills, coordination and endurance. For children with motor disabilities, active leisure activities in a setting adapted to their abilities help to develop their muscular strength, flexibility and balance, while promoting their independence. For example, a child in a wheelchair can take part in adapted sports such as wheelchair basketball or boccia, activities that not only improve their physical fitness, but also reinforce their ability to work as part of a team, respect rules and interact with others.

Leisure activities, particularly **group games,** are also a valuable tool for developing the **social skills** of disabled children. They offer them the opportunity to interact with their peers in a less formal environment than school, where children can learn to cooperate, resolve conflicts, share and understand others' points of view. For a child with a disability, these social interactions can sometimes be more difficult to establish in conventional school settings, where academic pressure or the rigid structure of classes can hinder the spontaneity of relationships. In leisure settings, the child is often more relaxed, more open to others, and has the opportunity to develop friendships based on shared interests rather than academic performance.

These moments of socialization are all the more important as they contribute to **the** child's **social inclusion**. Leisure activities offer a setting in which disability can be perceived not as a barrier, but as a particularity among others. When well supervised and inclusive, these moments enable children with disabilities to feel accepted and valued, and other children to develop a better understanding and acceptance of differences. For example, in artistic activities such as theater, painting or music, personal expression and creativity come to the fore, and disability becomes secondary. This type of leisure activity enables children to focus on their talents, rather than their limitations, and to forge bonds with their peers on the basis of shared experiences, reinforcing their sense of belonging and self-confidence.

The **emotional support** provided by leisure activities is also essential for disabled children. These activities enable them to escape the constraints often imposed by disability or the demands of everyday life. Whether through play, art, sport or outings, leisure activities offer children a space to express themselves freely, explore new interests and discover skills they never knew they had. For example, a child who takes part in an artistic activity, such as painting or sculpting, may find it an outlet for expressing emotions that he or she is not always able to verbalize. Leisure activities then become a means of exploring facets of his personality and boosting his self-esteem, by highlighting his successes and progress, rather than focusing solely on the obstacles linked to his disability.

Leisure activities are also a great opportunity **to stimulate** children's **imagination and creativity**. Artistic and cultural activities, such as music, dance, theater or visual arts, enable children to express themselves non-verbally and unleash their creativity, whatever their physical or cognitive ability. These activities are particularly important for children with communication disorders or difficulties expressing themselves verbally, as they offer them an alternative means of communication. For example, an autistic child can express himself through music or painting, using these mediums to share emotions or ideas that he can't put into words. These forms of artistic expression are liberating and enable the child to feel valued for his or her talents, rather than stigmatized by his or her disability.

What's more, leisure activities are an opportunity for children to **develop their autonomy**. By taking part in leisure activities, children learn to make decisions, manage their time and organize themselves in a playful, less structured setting than that of school or care. For example, a child who participates in an organized outing to the park or in a creative workshop may be encouraged to make his or her own choices, manage personal affairs, or take the initiative in interacting with peers. This kind of experience helps children to develop greater self-confidence and a sense of control over their environment, which is essential for their personal development and for the acquisition of skills that will be useful throughout their lives.

Finally, leisure activities can be a way of **changing the** way in **which** disability is **viewed**, both by the child and by those around him. By succeeding in a leisure activity, children show their parents, peers and the adults around them that they have skills and talents that go far beyond their disability. This helps redefine the child's self-image, as well as that of others. For example, a child who takes part in a dance show or an adapted sports competition shows that he or she is capable of succeeding and excelling in areas he or she is passionate about, while showcasing his or her abilities and stamina.

- **Adapt games and activities to specific needs**

Adapting games and activities to the specific needs of children with disabilities is an essential step towards their inclusion and development. Beyond their playful dimension, games are a powerful development tool, whether for learning, socializing or exploring the world. However, each child is unique, and his or her needs - be they physical, sensory or cognitive - often require adjustments to ensure that activities are fully accessible and beneficial. Adapting games doesn't simply mean making an activity doable, but enabling the child to participate in an active and rewarding way, while taking into account his or her individual skills and challenges. In this way, every child can engage in activities that stimulate their imagination, develop their social and motor skills, and boost their self-esteem.

**Adapting play equipment for children with motor disabilities** means first and foremost taking into account their physical abilities and mobility. Children with motor difficulties may need additional supports or physical adaptations to participate in activities. For example, for a child in a wheelchair, ball games or races can be adjusted by using lighter balls, lowering targets or organizing throwing activities rather than running. Group games, such as basketball or adapted field hockey, allow children to interact with their peers, while adjusting the rules so that everyone can participate fully. Similarly, specially designed equipment, such as accessible-wheelchair swings or harness systems for climbing activities, enable children to engage in physical play that would otherwise be inaccessible to them.

**Fine motor games** can also be adapted for children with limited use of their hands. Puzzles, construction games or manual activities can be adjusted by offering larger pieces, softer materials, or adapted tools. For example, if a child has difficulty grasping small objects, ergonomic brushes or pencils can be used to facilitate artistic activities. Building sets, such as LEGOs or blocks, can be adapted with larger pieces or more textured surfaces, making them easier to grip and reinforcing the child's independence in the activity.

For children with **sensory disorders**, such as visual or hearing impairments, adapting games often involves modifying the stimuli used. For a visually impaired or blind child, games must be based on auditory, tactile or olfactory stimuli. For example, a classic board game can be adapted with Braille or embossed pieces, and memory games can be redesigned using different textures, sound objects or elements to be identified by touch. For outdoor activities, such as races or treasure hunts, sound signals can be used to guide the child, enabling him or her to take an active part in the activity without feeling excluded. Deaf or hard-of-hearing children, meanwhile, will benefit from visual games, such as light, movement or mime games, where communication takes place through gestures, signs or images. Group activities can be enhanced by the use of sign language or pictograms, enabling fluid interaction between the child and his peers.

**Children with cognitive or learning disabilities**, such as dyslexia, dyscalculia or autism spectrum disorders, require games and activities adapted to their pace and way of understanding information. Games need to be structured, with clear instructions, simplified rules and well-defined stages. Children with autism, for example, may be more comfortable with games that follow predictable routines and offer a structured framework. Building, sorting or classifying activities are often very beneficial for these children, as they reinforce their sense of organization and logic while stimulating their concentration. For children with attention problems, games requiring short phases of activity, with integrated breaks, help maintain their interest while respecting their need to relax.

In creative activities such as painting, drawing or modeling, adaptation must also take account of each child's abilities. **Artistic activities** are often an excellent way for children with disabilities to express their creativity and emotions, while stimulating their sensory and motor development. For children with motor difficulties, adapted supports can be provided, such as adjustable easels or brushes with wider handles, making them easier to hold. Children with sensory difficulties, meanwhile, can thrive on multisensory activities, such as modeling with clay, finger-painting or exploring textured materials, which engage their sense of touch and help them explore their environment in a richer, more interactive way.

In **group play,** it's essential to adapt not only the activities, but also the attitude of the other participants. Raising awareness among the disabled child's peers is a fundamental step in creating an inclusive play environment. Other children need to be encouraged to participate in a caring way and to help their peers integrate into the activities, without over-protecting or unintentionally excluding them. For example, in a team game such as dodgeball, it is possible to adapt the rules to enable a child with physical limitations to participate actively, by offering opportunities to throw or aim differently. This type of adaptation shows that everyone can contribute to the activity in their own way, while reinforcing cohesion and mutual support within the group.

It's also important to remember that adapted games should enable the child to **develop his** or **her skills** while enjoying the activity. Adaptation should not mean oversimplifying the game, but rather adjusting the rules, tools or environment so that the child can participate fully, while being stimulated and encouraged to progress. For example, in an educational game such as Scrabble, a dyslexic child can use an enlarged board with more visible letters or illustrated cards, while continuing to play according to the same rules as the other children. This maintains the child's interest in the game, while helping them to overcome their difficulties.

Finally, **the role of the adult** is essential in adapting games and activities. Teachers, caregivers, care assistants and parents need to be attentive to the specific needs of each child, and propose adaptations without creating additional barriers or feelings of difference. The adult must play a supporting role, ensuring that the child participates actively and takes full advantage of the activities on offer. For example, during a creative workshop, the adult can encourage the child to explore different techniques, while offering supports adapted to the child's motor or sensory abilities. Similarly, in group games, the adult can modulate the rules to ensure that every child has the opportunity to participate equally, while respecting each child's individuality.

- **Facilitate integration into children's groups: outings, vacations**

Facilitating the integration of children with disabilities into groups of children, particularly during outings and vacations, is essential for their social development and emotional well-being. These moments outside the usual school or home environment are precious opportunities for discovery, sharing and learning. They enable children to experience new situations, strengthen their social skills, and forge bonds with their peers. However, for these experiences to be fully beneficial, it is important to provide adaptations and supervision tailored to the specific needs of each child, while fostering an inclusive and caring environment.

**School or group outings**, such as museum excursions, cultural visits or nature outings, are moments of collective discovery. For children with disabilities, these outings can present physical, sensory or cognitive challenges. It is therefore crucial to anticipate the child's specific needs to ensure that the experience is as positive as possible. This can include physical accessibility features, such as the use of adapted vehicles or the organization of a route without major obstacles. For example, if an outing involves a long walk, it may be necessary to plan regular breaks, shorter routes or allow the child to use a wheelchair if this facilitates participation. The aim is to enable the child to participate fully in the activity, without feeling excluded or limited by his or her disability.

In addition to physical adaptations, it's important to **prepare your child in advance of** the outing, especially if he or she is cognitively impaired or has difficulty managing transitions. Preparation helps to reduce anxiety and facilitate adaptation to a new environment. This can involve clear, simple explanations of what's going to happen on the outing, using visual aids or pictograms for children with communication difficulties. For example, for an outing to the zoo, pictures of the animals that the child will see, photos of the place, or a description of the different stages of the day can help the child to project himself and better understand what awaits him. This anticipation is particularly important for children with autism or anxiety disorders, who may be stressed by the unknown or changes in routine.

**Raising awareness among the group of children** is another key step in facilitating integration during outings or vacations. It's important that the other children understand the specific needs of their disabled peers, without stigmatizing them. This can be done in advance, by discussing with the group the diversity of abilities and the importance of mutual help and inclusion. For example, explaining to children that one of their peers needs more time to get around, or that he or she communicates differently, creates a climate of empathy and mutual respect. In this way, children learn to be attentive to the needs of others, while developing social skills such as listening, patience and cooperation.

**Group vacations**, such as summer camps, are unique opportunities for children to forge strong friendships, develop their independence and blossom in a different setting. For children with disabilities, these experiences are particularly important, as they provide an opportunity for fun and relaxation outside the daily routine, while reinforcing their social inclusion. However, to ensure that these vacations take place in the best possible conditions, it is necessary to provide specific supervision and activities adapted to their abilities. This can include instructors trained to accompany disabled children, diversified activities that take into account the children's physical or sensory limitations, or flexible schedules that respect each child's rhythm.

It's also important to encourage **the active participation of every child** on these group vacations. Rather than offering separate activities for children with disabilities, the ideal solution is to adapt activities so that they can include all children. For example, in a sporting activity such as soccer or swimming, it is possible to modulate the rules of the game or use specific equipment so that each child can participate in his or her own way. Children who can't run can be encouraged to throw or pass the ball, while those with sensory difficulties can benefit from individual coaching. This approach not only creates an inclusive dynamic, but also boosts the self-confidence of children with disabilities, who see their efforts and participation valued within the group.

**The organization of vacations and outings** must also take into account the medical or specific needs of children with disabilities. This can include the management of medication, special monitoring of certain health aspects, or even dietary adaptations in case of specific needs. For children with epilepsy, for example, it's important that instructors are trained to manage a seizure, while ensuring that the child doesn't feel stigmatized or restricted in his or her participation. Similarly, it's crucial that vacation and outing sites are chosen for their accessibility, safety and ability to accommodate children with special needs. A suitable environment enables the child to enjoy these moments in complete serenity, without his or her disability becoming an obstacle to personal development.

**Emotional** support is another key aspect of integration during outings and vacations. These moments, while joyful and enriching, can also be a source of stress or anxiety for some children with disabilities, particularly when it comes to leaving their usual surroundings or adapting to a group they don't yet know well. The caregiver must be attentive to these moments of fragility, offering reassuring and benevolent support. This can take the form of regular exchanges with the child to check how he or she is feeling, moments of relaxation or withdrawal if the child needs a break, or encouragement to gradually take part in activities. Creating a climate of trust enables children to feel secure, overcome their fears and meet others with greater ease.

Finally, **communication with parents** is essential to ensure successful integration during outings and vacations. Parents are often the first to know about their child's specific needs, and can provide invaluable information on the adaptations required. An open dialogue with parents helps to anticipate potential problems and establish an appropriate support framework. It also gives parents the reassurance of knowing that their child will be well looked after, and that he or she will be able to experience these moments in a positive way. For example, before a summer camp, it can be useful to meet with the parents to discuss the child's needs, the equipment to be provided, or the specific arrangements to be made.

•     **Organize sensory and cognitive stimulation activities**
Organizing sensory and cognitive stimulation activities for children, especially those with disabilities, is a key approach to fostering their overall development, well-being and fulfillment. These activities stimulate the senses, enhance cognitive abilities and support the acquisition of new skills in a fun and engaging way. Tailored to the specific needs of each child, sensory and cognitive activities offer a learning opportunity by exploiting different sensory channels, while promoting independence, concentration and social interaction.

**Sensory stimulation** aims to awaken and develop the various senses - touch, sight, hearing, smell and taste - to help children better understand and explore their environment. For children with disabilities, these activities can be particularly beneficial, enabling them to overcome certain sensory limitations, improve their perception of the world and adjust their reactions to stimuli.

For example, for a child with **sensory processing disorders** (often seen in children with autism or attention disorders), activities that promote sensation regulation can be introduced. These can include tactile games involving the manipulation of different textures such as sand, water, clay, or balls of different materials. The idea is to create an environment where the child can freely experiment with a variety of sensations, enjoying exploring and touching without feeling overwhelmed. Activities such as finger-painting, manipulating play dough or slime, or exploring natural materials like leaves, pebbles or shells, are particularly effective in stimulating touch while enabling children to develop their fine motor skills.

**Visual and auditory sensory play** is also essential for children with visual or hearing impairments, or for those who react strongly to sensory stimuli. For example, activities using colored lights, visual contrasts or luminous objects such as fiber-optic lamps can help capture a visually impaired child's attention or reinforce residual visual skills. For hearing-impaired children, musical and sound games can be adapted using vibrations or low frequencies, enabling them to feel the sound through their bodies. In addition, musical listening sessions or the discovery of a variety of sounds (bells, drums, soft percussion) can stimulate their auditory senses while providing a soothing aspect.

**Cognitive** activities, **on** the other hand, aim to stimulate intellectual abilities such as memory, attention, problem-solving and logical reasoning. These activities are crucial to strengthening the learning skills of children, especially those with cognitive impairments or attention disorders. They can be designed to be both stimulating and accessible, taking into account the particularities of each child.

For example, adapted **memory games**, such as visual or tactile memorys, are playful ways of strengthening children's short-term memory and ability to concentrate. For children with cognitive difficulties, games should be simple and clear, with recognizable and attractive images or objects. Raised cards can be used for children with visual impairments, or sounds associated with objects for those who are more sensitive to auditory stimuli.

**Logic and problem-solving games** can also be adapted to suit children's abilities. Simplified puzzles, sorting or association games, or mazes can be used to encourage thinking and decision-making. The aim is to provide cognitive challenges within the reach of every child, while enabling them to progress at their own pace. For children who have difficulty concentrating or understanding complex instructions, instructions can be simplified and broken down into small steps, with positive reinforcement for each success.

**Integrating both types of stimulation - sensory and cognitive -** into a single activity can also be particularly beneficial. For example, simple cooking workshops combine sensory aspects (touching food, smelling odors, tasting) with cognitive skills (following a recipe, measuring quantities, waiting for the result). This type of activity offers a multisensory experience while reinforcing the cognitive skills of planning, attention and memory. Likewise, artistic activities such as painting, sculpting or modelling can stimulate concentration and imagination, while stimulating the senses. These experiences enable children to engage fully in the creative process while working on their intellectual and sensory skills.

For children with more complex disorders, such as **autism spectrum disorders** or **multiple disabilities**, snoezelen sessions can be set up. This multi-sensory space, designed to provide a calm yet stimulating environment, enables work on both relaxation and sensory stimulation, using soft lighting, varied textures, soothing sounds and pleasant smells. Children can explore at their own pace, without pressure, choosing stimuli that appeal to them and promote their well-being.

Another example of an activity combining **sensory and cognitive stimulation** might be an adapted treasure hunt. In this activity, the child is encouraged to solve simple clues or follow sensory trails to find hidden objects. The clues can be adapted according to the child's abilities: objects to touch for visually impaired children, visual clues for those who need support in developing their cognitive skills, or sound clues for noise-sensitive children. This activity not only stimulates thinking and decision-making, but also engages the senses while having fun.

**The importance of adaptability** in the organization of activities should not be underestimated. Every child has his or her own abilities and limitations, and it's essential that activities are flexible enough to adjust to their specific needs. This may include pauses to allow the child to refocus, or adjustments in the duration of activities to avoid sensory or cognitive overload. Similarly, it's important that professionals - whether teachers, caregivers or AVSs - listen to the child and constantly adapt their approach to his or her reactions.

- **Working with specialist educators to promote inclusion**

Working with special educators to promote the inclusion of children with disabilities is a key approach that requires close collaboration, shared skills and a deep understanding of each child's specific needs. Inclusion aims to integrate children into social and educational environments where they can develop to the full, taking part in the same activities as their peers, while benefiting from appropriate support. Specialized educators play a fundamental role in this process, as they have invaluable expertise in supporting children with developmental disorders, learning difficulties or physical disabilities. By working hand in hand with them, caregivers, teachers and other health professionals can ensure that the child benefits from comprehensive, coherent and personalized support, guaranteeing his or her inclusion and fulfillment.

**One of the first aspects of working with special educators** is to establish fluid, regular communication. Specialized educators often have in-depth knowledge of the child's specific needs, skills and difficulties, and of the educational strategies that work best for him or her. Regular exchanges with them make it possible to adapt support methods to the child's progress, adjust activities in line with his or her evolution, and identify situations where further adaptations are required. For example, for a child with behavioral problems, the specialized educator can advise on specific approaches to managing moments of frustration or agitation, proposing decompression techniques or arrangements to encourage calm and concentration. This collaboration enables each professional to intervene coherently and harmoniously, while ensuring continuous monitoring of the child's progress.

**The implementation of adapted educational strategies** is another essential aspect of this collaboration. Specialized educators are trained to develop pedagogical and behavioral strategies that meet the needs of children with disabilities, while taking into account their pace and learning style. For example, for a child with autism who has difficulty understanding social interactions, the specialized educator may suggest role-playing or social scenarios that help the child better apprehend everyday situations. These tools enable the child to gradually develop social skills, while reinforcing his or her autonomy and self-confidence. Working with the educator, other professionals, such as teachers or caregivers, can integrate these strategies into the child's daily life, whether in the classroom, during group activities or during moments of relaxation.

**Adapting group activities** is also a priority when working with specialist educators. Inclusion means not only that the child is physically present in a group, but also that he or she actively participates in the activities in a rewarding way. To achieve this, it is often necessary to adjust activities to suit the child's abilities and needs. For example, in an artistic workshop or sporting activity, the specialized educator may suggest alternatives or specific supports to enable the child to express himself and develop fully. This may include the use of visual aids for a child with communication difficulties, or the creation of a quiet space for a child who is sensitive to noise. By collaborating with the educator, other team members can ensure that the child is fully integrated into the activity, without his or her special needs being an obstacle to participation.

**The special educator's role as mediator** in interactions with other children is also crucial to inclusion. Other children often don't understand the needs or behaviors of a peer with a disability, which can lead to misunderstanding and even exclusion. The special educator can intervene by explaining to the other children, in an age-appropriate way, the specific features of their playmate, and showing them how to include him or her in their games or activities. For example, for a child with language difficulties, the educator can teach his or her peers the importance of patience and listening, while showing them ways of communicating simply and effectively. This mediation work helps create a more inclusive and empathetic environment, where every child feels accepted and supported.

**Ongoing training for other professionals** is another fundamental aspect of working with special educators. Because of their expertise, they are often in a position to train or sensitize other professionals who interact with the child. This training can cover a wide range of subjects, such as behavior management techniques, pedagogical approaches adapted to learning disabilities, or alternative communication tools. By training teachers, care assistants and organizers in the specificities of disability, the specialized educator helps to reinforce the quality of overall support, while ensuring that the child benefits from consistent support, regardless of who is looking after him or her. For example, a specialized educator can train a team in the use of Makaton (a language of signs and symbols) to help a child communicate more easily in class or in group activities.

**The implementation of personalized educational projects** (PEP or PPS) is another area in which collaboration with the specialized educator is essential. These projects are designed to meet the child's specific needs and to ensure that all necessary adaptations are in place, whether in terms of timetabling, teaching methods or individual support. The special educator, in collaboration with teachers, parents and other professionals, plays a central role in developing and monitoring these projects. He or she ensures that each objective is realistic and achievable, while making sure that the child progresses in a secure and caring environment. This personalized follow-up enables the educational project to be adjusted as the child evolves, taking into account his successes and new skills, as well as any obstacles he may encounter.

Finally, **family support** is an essential component of collaboration with special educators. The parents of a child with a disability can sometimes feel helpless in the face of the challenges faced by their child, and the specialized educator, in partnership with other professionals, plays a key role in guiding and accompanying them. This can include practical advice on how to manage behavior at home, information on rights and available aid, or moments of exchange to help them better understand their child's needs. The specialized educator can also act as a link between the family and the school, ensuring that parents are fully involved in their child's educational journey and kept informed of progress. This all-round support reinforces the coherence between the different environments in which the child lives, while offering parents a place where they can be listened to and advised.

# 9.

# Social inclusion and the fight against stigmatization

- **Raising awareness of the need to accept differences**

Raising awareness of the need to accept differences is an essential step towards creating a more inclusive, caring society that respects everyone's particularities. Acceptance of difference, particularly that of children with disabilities, cannot be fully achieved without a collective effort to raise awareness, starting with education, understanding and empathy. Whether in a family, school, professional or social context, it is essential to promote a culture in which diversity is perceived as an asset, not an obstacle. Raising awareness among those around us helps to deconstruct prejudices, reduce fears of the unknown, and reinforce the idea that each individual, with his or her differences, has a unique value to contribute.

**One of the first aspects of awareness-raising** is to **educate those around us** about the nature of disabilities and the specific challenges faced by children with disabilities. All too often, exclusionary or rejecting behavior is the result of ignorance or deep-seated stereotypes. For example, children with autism, whose behavior can be misinterpreted, may be perceived as distant or aggressive by their peers, simply because their mode of communication is different. Raising awareness means explaining the peculiarities of these behaviors, making it clear that they are not "abnormal", but that they respond to a different functioning of the brain or body. Open discussions, training or workshops on different types of disability can help families, teachers, peers and the community to acquire the knowledge they need to better understand and accept these differences.

At school, for example, it's crucial to **make children aware** of the diversity of their abilities from **an early age**. Education about difference can start with adapted reading, classroom discussions, or games that promote inclusion. Talking about difference in a positive way, highlighting the specific skills and talents of children with disabilities, helps change the way other children look at their peers. These discussions can also help answer the natural questions that children ask themselves when confronted with behaviors or needs they don't understand. Explain to them, for example, that a visually impaired child can use specific tools to read, or that a child with autism spectrum disorders may need quiet time to concentrate better. The idea is to play down these differences and encourage an attitude of empathy and benevolence from an early age.

**The role of adults in raising awareness** is also crucial. Parents, teachers, caregivers, educators and healthcare professionals need to model acceptance and respect for diversity. Children learn by example, and they are greatly influenced by the attitudes of the adults around them. If an adult expresses embarrassment or discomfort about a difference, children are likely to reproduce that attitude. Conversely, when adults adopt a posture of openness, benevolent curiosity and welcoming of differences, children are more inclined to do the same. For example, a teacher who includes a disabled child in all class activities, while ensuring that his or her specific needs are respected, sends a strong message to other students: everyone has a place and deserves to be treated with respect and dignity.

**Raising awareness within families** is also essential. Parents of children with disabilities, as well as those of children without disabilities, need to be supported in this process of understanding and acceptance. For some parents, their child's disability can be a source of fear or misunderstanding, particularly if they lack the resources or information they need to understand the situation. That's why it's so important to provide them with forums for exchange and support, where they can share their experiences, ask questions and find answers to their concerns. Raising families' awareness also means encouraging them to approach difference in a positive way with their children, valuing skills and highlighting successes rather than limitations. This approach boosts the self-esteem of children with disabilities, and encourages their integration into the family and the community.

**Open communication and dialogue** are powerful tools for promoting acceptance of difference. All too often, misunderstandings or judgments arise from a lack of information or fear of doing the wrong thing. It's important to create spaces for dialogue, where everyone can ask questions without fear of being judged, and where answers are given with kindness and pedagogy. For example, a teacher can organize class discussions where pupils are invited to ask questions about disability, or a parent can encourage their children to talk about their emotions in the face of difference. This kind of open dialogue lifts taboos and fosters mutual understanding.

**Public awareness campaigns** are also an effective way of reaching a wider audience and changing attitudes on a large scale. These campaigns can take many forms: educational videos, testimonials from people with disabilities, workshops in schools, or community events celebrating diversity. These initiatives help to create a culture where difference is valued and stereotypes are deconstructed. For example, a campaign that highlights the achievements and talents of children with disabilities, whether in the arts, sports or school activities, can have a profound impact by showing that disability is not a limitation, but a particularity in its own right.

It is also essential to **promote a positive vision of difference**. All too often, difference - and disability in particular - is seen in a negative light, as an absence or a lack. This vision must be reversed to recognize that the diversity of abilities and functions enriches our society and teaches us to be more open and adaptable. Making those around us aware of this idea means encouraging a perspective in which each individual, with his or her strengths and weaknesses, contributes to the richness of the community. This means recognizing the achievements of children with disabilities, highlighting their talents, and encouraging them to be treated as equals, with specific rights and needs, but also with unique abilities.

**Actively including children in all activities** is also a powerful way of raising awareness of the need to accept differences. When a child with a disability takes part in a sporting, artistic or school activity alongside his or her peers, they demonstrate that they can integrate and flourish, provided that the necessary adaptations are put in place. This visible inclusion deconstructs prejudice and shows that, despite their differences, all children can share common experiences and learn from each other. For example, including a wheelchair-bound child in an adapted basketball team shows that participation is possible with simple accommodations, while reinforcing the group's sense of belonging.

- **Combating prejudice: the role of the caregiver in raising awareness**

Combating prejudice against people with disabilities is fundamental to building an inclusive society that respects differences and is open to diversity. Prejudice, often stemming from ignorance, fear or stereotypes, can create invisible barriers that isolate disabled children, affect their self-esteem and hinder their social integration. In this fight against preconceived ideas, the caregiver plays a key role as a health professional, accompanying these children on a daily basis. His or her work is not limited to providing physical care, but also includes an educational and social dimension, aimed at raising awareness among those around him or her of the need to accept differences and value the child's abilities. Through direct action and interaction with families, teachers and other children, the caregiver helps to deconstruct stereotypes and promote a positive, realistic view of disability.

**Fighting prejudice means first and foremost deconstructing stereotypes** that are deeply rooted in society. Disability is often perceived through a negative prism, associating the disabled person with an image of weakness, incapacity or total dependence. These misconceptions can influence the behavior of other children, adults and teachers, who, out of ignorance or fear of doing the wrong thing, may adopt an overprotective or even exclusionary attitude. The caregiver, by virtue of his or her position of proximity to the child, is well placed to show that these stereotypes are unfounded. He or she can, for example, encourage teachers and classmates to see the child's skills beyond his or her disability, highlighting his or her progress, talents and successes, even if these are not always manifested in conventional ways. Through daily actions and regular exchanges with those around them, the caregiver helps to change perceptions and show that every child, whatever his or her disability, has abilities to be valued.

**One of the caregivers' main missions in the fight against prejudice** is to inform and raise awareness among the child's direct entourage, in particular parents and family. Sometimes, the first prejudices arise within the family unit itself, where disability may be misunderstood or badly experienced. Some parents may find it hard to accept their child's disability, or may adopt an overprotective attitude that unintentionally limits the child's development. The caregiver's role of accompaniment and support can help families better understand their child's abilities, and adjust their expectations realistically. By explaining the child's potential, and showing them how he or she can progress with the right tools and support, the caregiver enables parents to review their perception of disability and better support their child's progress.

**In the school setting**, the caregiver also plays a key role in raising awareness among teachers and other students. School, as a place of socialization and learning, can also be a place where prejudices are born or reinforced, particularly when teachers or students don't know how to interact with a disabled child. For example, a child with behavioral problems or communication difficulties may be misperceived by peers who don't understand his or her reactions or specific needs. The caregiver, in collaboration with specialized educators and teachers, can help to explain the child's particularities in a simple, accessible way, and suggest strategies to promote inclusion. They can also teach other children the importance of mutual support, respect and tolerance. Organizing class discussions or inclusive games is a concrete way of showing students that difference is no obstacle to friendship or cooperation.

**Valuing children's abilities** is another essential aspect of the fight against prejudice. One of the greatest challenges facing children with disabilities is the way they are viewed by others. Often, they are reduced to their disability, their limitations highlighted, while their skills or talents go unnoticed. The caregiver can help change this perception by highlighting the child's successes, both large and small. For example, he or she can encourage the child to take part in group activities, even with adaptations, and to show off his or her skills in areas where he or she excels, such as art, music or adapted sports. This kind of encouragement not only boosts the child's self-esteem, but also changes the way others look at him/her, as they begin to see beyond the disability.

**The** caregiver's **emotional support** for the child is also crucial in the fight against prejudice. Children with disabilities can sometimes internalize stereotypes or negative ideas that others have of them, which can affect their self-confidence and willingness to take part in activities. By listening attentively and providing daily support, the caregiver can help the child develop a positive self-image, become aware of his or her skills and feel valued. This involves words of encouragement, congratulations for every step forward, and the establishment of a trusting relationship in which the child feels supported and understood. By strengthening the child's self-confidence, the caregiver gives him or her the tools needed to face up to outside scrutiny and judgment, while enabling him or her to assert him or herself and participate fully in social life.

**The caregiver's role does not stop at raising awareness of others**, it also includes a mediation dimension. They may be called upon to intervene in situations where prejudice or misunderstanding create tension or conflict. For example, if a disabled child is ostracized or teased by his or her classmates, the caregiver can act as a mediator to explain the situation, defuse misunderstandings and propose solutions to reintegrate the child into the group. This mediation not only resolves immediate conflicts, but also creates a more positive long-term dynamic, where children learn to accept differences and interact respectfully.

**Ongoing training** is another important lever in the fight against prejudice. As healthcare professionals, caregivers must themselves be trained in the various forms of disability, in communication and inclusion strategies, and in techniques for raising awareness among others. By keeping up to date with best practice and sharing their knowledge with colleagues, families and the community, carers help to create a more inclusive and informed environment. What's more, by networking with other professionals, such as specialist educators, psychologists or teachers, they can reinforce the effectiveness of their action and ensure that awareness-raising is carried out in a coherent, concerted manner.

- **Encouraging children to develop positive self-esteem**

Encouraging children, especially those with disabilities, to develop positive self-esteem is a fundamental task that influences their well-being, their ability to face life's challenges and their social integration. Self-esteem is a child's perception of his or her own worth, skills and ability to be loved and accepted. For a child with a disability, this perception can sometimes be put to the test by the difficulties he or she encounters, the way others look at him or her, or the physical or cognitive limitations he or she has to overcome. In this context, the caregiver, in liaison with the child's parents, teachers and entourage, plays a key role in enabling the child to build a positive self-image, based on his or her successes and strengths, and not just on his or her difficulties.

**The first essential element** in **fostering positive self-esteem** is to focus on the child's **strengths and abilities,** rather than his or her limitations. Too often, children with disabilities are perceived through the prism of what they cannot do, rather than what they can achieve. The caregiver, through his or her daily accompaniment, can show the child that his or her abilities are real and deserve to be valued. For example, a child with motor difficulties who is gifted at drawing should be encouraged to develop his artistic skills, to take part in activities where he can express his talent, and to see this skill as a source of pride. It's essential to congratulate the child on every small success, no matter how insignificant it may seem. Every step forward, every effort counts in building positive self-esteem. Children need to feel that their efforts are recognized and that they are capable of learning, improving and succeeding, at their own pace and according to their own abilities.

**Valuing successes**, however small, is a powerful motor for boosting self-esteem. For a child with a disability, certain tasks may require more effort or time than their peers, which can lead to discouragement or feelings of inferiority. The caregiver can counter this by celebrating small victories and focusing on progress rather than immediate performance. For example, if a child achieves even a small goal, such as writing a few letters or actively participating in a group activity, it's important to acknowledge this accomplishment. Positive reinforcement helps children understand that their efforts are meaningful and that they can overcome obstacles with perseverance.

At the same time, it's crucial to **avoid comparisons**. Each child develops at his or her own pace and under specific conditions. Comparisons with other children, especially those without disabilities, can be destructive and seriously damage the child's self-esteem. The caregiver, like the other adults in the child's life, must be careful to value the child's achievements without comparing them to those of his or her peers. The emphasis should be on the child's personal progress, showing that each journey is unique and that successes are important in themselves, without the need to measure them against those of others.

**Developing children's autonomy** is also an important lever for boosting their self-esteem. The more a child is able to accomplish tasks on his own, the more confidence he gains in his abilities. The caregiver can, on a daily basis, encourage the child to take part in activities adapted to his or her level, guiding him or her while leaving him or her free to do things on his or her own. For example, a child can be encouraged to dress himself, prepare a simple snack or choose the activities he wants to do. Even if it takes longer, or if the child needs a little help, it's essential to give him the opportunity to develop his autonomy. Seeing that he can accomplish tasks independently reinforces his sense of competence and, consequently, his self-confidence.

**Listening to and respecting the child's emotions** are also central to fostering positive self-esteem. It's important for children to feel heard and understood in their day-to-day lives, especially when they encounter difficulties or frustrations. The caregiver's supportive role can provide a safe space for the child to express fears, disappointments or anger. Acknowledging these emotions without judgment enables the child to understand that his feelings are legitimate and that he has the right to experience moments of weakness, without this affecting his worth. For example, if a child fails at a task he was hoping to succeed at, it's essential to help him accept this failure, while encouraging him to persevere. This shows him that failure is part of learning and does not call into question his abilities.

The child's social environment - whether family, school or outside activities - also plays a decisive role in building self-esteem. **Encouraging the child's social integration** is an effective way of helping him feel valued by others and reinforcing his sense of belonging. The caregiver can encourage the child to participate in group activities, interact with peers, and feel included in social life. For example, by adapting group games or facilitating communication with other children, the caregiver enables the child to participate actively and feel accepted by others. This sense of belonging is fundamental to the child building a positive self-image, seeing himself or herself as a full member of the group, rather than as someone "different".

Finally, **the language used** around the child is an important element in building self-esteem. It's crucial to use language that is both positive and caring, avoiding terms that might reduce the child to his or her disability or give the impression that he or she is "incapable". Talking to the child about his successes, encouraging him to try new things, and using positive, constructive phrases all help to reinforce his self-image. For example, instead of saying "You can't do that because of your disability", it's better to say "You can try it this way, and I'll help you get there". This positive approach enables the child to focus on what he can achieve, rather than on what is difficult for him.

# 10.

# Supporting the transition to adolescence and adulthood

- **Understanding the challenges of puberty in children with disabilities**

Puberty is a crucial stage of development for all children, marked by significant physical, emotional and psychological changes. For children with disabilities, this period can present additional challenges, as the transformations that accompany puberty can interact in complex ways with the particularities associated with their disability. Understanding these challenges is essential to providing adequate, respectful and caring support to these children, while helping them to get through this delicate period as serenely as possible.

**The physical changes of puberty**, such as rapid growth and the development of secondary sexual characteristics (such as the appearance of breasts in girls or body hair in boys), can be confusing and even frightening for some children with disabilities, especially those with cognitive impairments or difficulties in understanding these transformations. For a child with an intellectual disability, for example, it can be difficult to grasp the normality of these changes, which can generate confusion, anxiety or even distress. One of the first challenges for parents, caregivers and educators is to help the child understand these bodily changes. This can be done through simple explanations, adapted to the child's level of understanding, using visual aids or educational tools designed to make this information accessible. It's important to show the child that these changes are natural and not linked to an illness or problem.

**The hormonal transformations** that occur during puberty can also influence a child's behavior and emotions. Mood swings, irritability and heightened sensitivity are common phenomena in teenagers, but in children with disabilities, these manifestations can be amplified or made more difficult to manage. For example, an autistic child, already sensitive to external stimuli, may feel even more intensely the emotional upheavals induced by hormones. It is therefore crucial to provide a calm, structured environment where the child feels secure, while giving him/her the tools to express his/her emotions appropriately. Caregivers and parents need to be attentive to these changes, and ensure that the child has spaces to release stress, such as moments of relaxation, meditation or soothing activities.

Another complex aspect of puberty for disabled children is **the management of personal hygiene**. With puberty come changes such as increased sweating, the appearance of acne, or the management of menstruation in girls. For a child with motor difficulties or an intellectual disability, these aspects can be a source of frustration or embarrassment, as it can be difficult for them to maintain adequate hygiene without help. One of the challenges for parents and caregivers is to find the right balance between encouraging autonomy and providing the necessary assistance. For example, a child with motor difficulties may need technical aids, such as special handles for using the shower, or guidance in learning personal hygiene gestures. For girls having their first period, it's crucial to prepare them for this moment by explaining what's going to happen and helping them understand how to deal with this new reality in a practical, panic-free way.

In addition to the physical and emotional challenges, **puberty also raises questions about sexuality**, a subject often complex to broach with children, and even more so when they have a disability. Sexuality is part of human development, but it can be surrounded by taboos, fears or misunderstandings, especially for children with cognitive disorders. It's essential to treat this subject with sensitivity, but also in a clear and informative way. Disabled children, like all others, need to receive sexuality education that corresponds to their mental age and capacity for understanding. This can include information about relationships, consent and bodily changes, as well as the importance of respecting one's own body and that of others. The challenge here is twofold: to help children understand and accept the transformations they are going through, and to give them the keys to navigating complex social situations where issues of interpersonal relationships or sexuality may arise.

**Social interactions** often become more complicated at puberty, as teenagers seek to define themselves within groups and develop relationships with their peers. For children with disabilities, this quest for identity and acceptance can be particularly difficult. The gaze of others, often marked by prejudice or misunderstanding, can exacerbate feelings of difference and rejection. It is therefore essential to help children develop positive self-esteem and confidence in their abilities, despite the difficulties they may encounter in their social relationships. The caregiver, in conjunction with teachers and parents, can play a crucial role in helping the child find ways to express himself and interact with his peers, while offering emotional support to cope with any frustrations or rejections.

Another challenge concerns **the perception of autonomy** among adolescents with disabilities. At puberty, many children aspire to greater independence, whether in the management of their bodies, in their choice of clothing, or in their daily activities. However, for children with disabilities, this quest for autonomy may come up against physical or cognitive limitations that make it difficult to achieve this goal. For example, a child with motor difficulties may wish to dress himself or take part in sporting activities, but may feel frustrated by his inability to perform these tasks without help. It's important to support the child's aspirations to autonomy, while helping him to recognize his limits without negatively affecting his self-esteem. This means encouraging them to try things out, adapting their environment to encourage this autonomy, and providing caring support that respects the child's rhythm.

**Support from parents and professionals** is crucial in helping children navigate through the challenges of puberty. It's important for parents to be informed and supported in this process, as they themselves may feel helpless in the face of their child's transformations. The caregiver, as a privileged interlocutor, can offer practical advice on how to approach these changes, on sexuality education, or even on managing the new responsibilities linked to bodily hygiene. The support of healthcare professionals, such as doctors or psychologists, may also be needed to manage certain specific aspects, such as hormonal disorders, mood changes or behavioral difficulties that can accompany puberty.

- **Supporting young people through physical and emotional changes**

Accompanying young people as they go through physical and emotional changes is a major challenge, requiring both a detailed understanding of the transformations they are going through, and tailored support to help them live through this transitional period with serenity and confidence. These changes, which occur mainly at puberty, mark a crucial stage in human development. They affect not only the body, but also emotions, self-image and the way young people perceive and interact with the world. For some, these are transformations a source of enthusiasm and excitement, while for others they can be experienced with anxiety, confusion or unease. The support of adults, whether parents, educators, teachers or caregivers, is therefore fundamental in guiding young people through this delicate phase, providing them with the tools and support they need to better understand and accept what they are experiencing.

**The bodily changes** associated with puberty, such as rapid growth, the appearance of secondary sexual characteristics, or the change in a boy's voice, can upset a young person's self-image. These sometimes spectacular and rapid transformations can be experienced with curiosity, but also with apprehension. Some young people may feel uncomfortable with their new bodies, especially if these changes do not occur at the same pace as their peers. In such cases, it's crucial to explain that puberty is a normal and universal stage, which unfolds differently for each individual. This support should be accompanied by open discussions about the changes to come, to help young people better anticipate them. For example, it's important to talk to girls about menstruation before it happens, so they aren't surprised or worried. Similarly, boys need to be prepared for vocal changes or the appearance of body hair. The language used should be simple, caring and age-appropriate, to reassure them and give them confidence in this natural process.

**Hygiene management** is an essential dimension of this support. With puberty, the body changes and new responsibilities arise in terms of personal care: sweating becomes more marked, the appearance of acne may require specific care, and girls must learn to manage their first periods. Many young people may feel embarrassed or uncomfortable in the face of these new realities. So it's essential to teach them, without judgment, how to care for their bodies in light of these changes. For example, it's important to explain why it's necessary to wash more regularly, change clothes or use deodorant, while providing practical advice on how to manage these new aspects of body hygiene. This learning process should not be experienced as a constraint, but as a way of taking care of oneself and feeling good about one's changing body.

**On an emotional level**, puberty is also a time of upheaval. Hormones, in full effervescence, cause mood swings, moments of heightened sensitivity, even irritability or sadness. Young people may find it difficult to understand or control these emotions, which can destabilize them. They may feel lost, misunderstood or overwhelmed by feelings they don't always know how to express. Adult support is therefore essential to help them through these moments. It's important to make them understand that these emotions are normal and part of the maturing process. Active listening is essential: young people must be allowed to express their feelings freely, without minimizing or judging them. For example, if a teenager feels sad or angry for no apparent reason, it's important to tell him or her that this is a normal, temporary reaction, while suggesting strategies for managing these emotions, such as taking part in a relaxing or sporting activity.

**Building self-esteem** is also a key aspect of this support. With body and emotional changes, a young person's self-image can be profoundly affected. Some may feel less sure of themselves, while others may suffer from complexes linked to their physical appearance or social performance. This is the time when the gaze of others, especially peers, becomes particularly important, and can significantly influence self-esteem. Even trivial remarks can have a profound impact on the way young people perceive themselves. For this reason, it's essential that adults encourage positive body and self-image. They need to value young people's strengths and qualities, beyond the physical, by highlighting their skills, efforts and successes. By helping them to understand that each body is unique and that diversity of appearance is a source of richness, we help them to build a solid self-esteem, capable of withstanding social pressures.

**Social relationships**, especially friendships and love affairs, take center stage during puberty. Young people seek to integrate into groups, to be accepted, and often begin to experience romantic feelings. These new experiences can be a source of joy, but also of concern, especially when they are not shared or when they lead to questions about their own identity. Accompanying young people in this area is essential, in particular to help them understand the notions of consent, mutual respect and personal limits. It's crucial to explain to them that relationships, whether friendly or romantic, must be based on reciprocity, benevolence and respect for differences. Adults must be available to answer the sometimes delicate questions that young people ask themselves at this stage of their lives, without judgment or embarrassment.

**Helping young people through puberty also means providing them with appropriate sex education**. Puberty is often the period when the first questions about sexuality emerge. It's vital to provide them with clear, objective information on how their bodies work, sexual relationships and the issues surrounding contraception and protection against sexually transmitted diseases. These discussions must be conducted in a caring manner, in a setting where young people feel confident to ask questions. It's also important to address the emotional dimension of sexuality, insisting on respect for oneself and others, and explaining that each individual has the right to decide about his or her own body and relationships. Sexuality education, properly understood and adapted to the age of young people, is a powerful way of helping them to take responsibility and feel comfortable with their bodies and their choices.

Finally, **the role of adults,** whether parents, teachers, caregivers or educators, is to accompany young people while giving them space to explore their identity and emotions. It's essential to create a climate of trust, where young people know they can talk freely about their doubts and concerns. Adults must be available, attentive and open to dialogue, while respecting the teenager's privacy and need for independence. By fostering this relationship of trust, they enable young people to get through this period of upheaval with greater serenity and confidence.

- **Preparing for independence: autonomy in personal care**

Preparing young people, especially those with disabilities, for independence by developing their self-care skills is a crucial step on their path to a fulfilling adult life. The acquisition of these skills is essential not only to boost their self-confidence, but also to enable them to participate actively in their daily lives and their environment. Developing autonomy in personal care - be it hygiene, dressing, managing bodily needs or making health-related decisions - is a gradual process that requires patience, pedagogy and caring support. Each young person, according to his or her abilities and challenges, can develop these skills at his or her own pace, with the support of caregivers, parents and educators.

**One of the first aspects of preparing for independence** is **learning the basics of daily hygiene**. Washing, brushing one's teeth, caring for one's skin and styling one's hair are essential tasks which, when mastered, give the child or teenager a sense of control and pride. For children with motor or cognitive difficulties, these gestures may require specific adaptations. For example, a child with difficulty holding a toothbrush may need a wider handle or an electric toothbrush. The caregiver, in collaboration with the parents, can help identify the appropriate tools and teach the child the essential gestures gradually. It's important to break tasks down into simple, repeated steps, so that the child can gradually integrate these routines. Constant encouragement and recognition of progress, however modest, are essential to boost motivation and self-esteem.

Autonomy in personal care also **means learning to manage clothing**. Dressing oneself, choosing clothes to suit the climate or circumstances, learning to tie shoelaces or button a coat are all important steps towards independence. For some children, these gestures may seem complex or frustrating. So it's essential to teach them these skills using appropriate teaching aids. For example, clothes with simpler fastenings, such as velcro or press-studs, can make learning easier. The caregiver can also guide the child through these steps, showing him or her how to proceed step by step. This process should be gradual, respecting the child's pace and allowing time for experimentation and error. Autonomy in dressing is not only a practical skill, it also enables children to develop their identity, make personal choices, and feel more in control of their daily lives.

**Managing bodily needs**, such as going to the toilet or changing one's sanitary protection, represents another major challenge in the acquisition of independence. For young people, especially those with disabilities, these acts can be a source of anxiety or embarrassment. It's crucial to approach them delicately and in a way that doesn't dramatize them. Learning to use the toilet should be a gradual process, involving the provision of clear guidelines, such as regular toilet times, and adapting the environment to make it more accessible (adapted toilets, grab bars, etc.). The caregiver can also help establish a routine for these gestures, enabling the child to feel more confident and to integrate these practices as normal steps in daily life. For girls, the management of menstruation is a delicate aspect that requires specific education, but also support so that they can manage this moment independently, without stress or discomfort.

**Taking care of one's health** is another essential component of autonomy. Young people must gradually learn to listen to their bodies, understand their needs, and make health-related decisions. This can include simple gestures such as staying sufficiently hydrated, recognizing signs of fatigue, or managing minor injuries. For some children with chronic conditions or specific medical needs, acquiring autonomy also involves managing their treatments. For example, a diabetic child can learn, with the support of his caregivers, to measure his blood sugar levels, recognize the symptoms of hypoglycemia, or administer his own treatment under supervision. This is a gradual process, depending on the child's maturity and abilities, but it is crucial for building confidence in one's own abilities and for preparing the transition to adulthood.

As part of this learning process, the caregiver must also **create an encouraging and respectful environment**, where the child feels supported, but also empowered. It's essential to give the child the space to try things out for him/herself, while remaining present to support him/her in case of difficulty. For example, rather than always performing care on the child's behalf, the caregiver can suggest that he or she perform certain gestures alone, under benevolent supervision. By letting the child experiment, even if it takes time or if the result is not perfect, we enable him or her to gradually acquire skills while building self-confidence.

It is also essential **not to overprotect** the child in the process of learning autonomy. The temptation can be great, especially for parents or carers, to do things for the child to save time or avoid mistakes. However, this approach can hinder the development of independence. Autonomy is not built by avoiding difficulties, but by enabling the child to face them with appropriate support. It's important to understand that learning to be independent is a process that involves trial and error, but that these mistakes are normal and necessary steps towards self-mastery.

Finally, **emotional support** plays a key role in preparing the child for independence. The acquisition of new skills, particularly in the field of personal care, can sometimes generate frustration or fear of failure in the child. So it's important that the caregiver listens to the child's emotions, encourages him or her to persevere, and values every effort, even if the result isn't perfect. For example, if a child has difficulty brushing his teeth properly, the caregiver can show him the correct technique while praising his attempts. This approach boosts the child's motivation and shows him that he is capable of learning, even if it takes time.

- **Working with families to plan long-term care**

Collaborating with families to plan long-term care is a fundamental aspect of supporting children with disabilities or complex medical needs. This collaboration aims to put in place sustainable, adapted and flexible strategies to meet the child's needs throughout his or her life. Long-term care planning is not just about the medical aspects, but also encompasses the child's emotional, social and educational well-being. Families play a central role in this process, as they are often the first to understand their child's specific needs and to anticipate future challenges. Working in partnership with them enables us to build a care plan that takes into account the day-to-day realities of the child and his or her family, while drawing on the expertise of healthcare professionals, educators and caregivers.

**The first step in working successfully with families** is to establish a climate of trust. It is essential that parents feel listened to, respected and understood. Long-term care planning can be a source of anxiety for families, as it involves anticipating the future and taking potentially difficult situations into account. It is therefore crucial that parents can express their concerns, expectations and wishes for their child's future without feeling judged. The caregiver, as the professional on hand, plays a key role in this dialogue. He or she must be an active listener, taking the time to understand the child's needs in the context of his or her family, while offering practical, realistic advice based on his or her expertise.

**The active involvement of parents in decision-making** is also a central pillar of this collaboration. Long-term care planning should not be imposed, but built in partnership with the family. Each family has its own priorities, values and dynamics, which must be respected and taken into account in the development of the care plan. For example, some parents may wish their child to be cared for at home for as long as possible, while others may envisage specialized structures adapted to their child's complex needs. It's important to engage in an open discussion about different care options, clearly outlining the advantages and disadvantages of each solution, while respecting families' choices. This collaborative approach ensures that the decisions taken truly reflect the family's needs and aspirations.

**Coordination is** another key aspect of long-term care planning. Children with disabilities are often cared for by a multi-disciplinary team, including doctors, nurses, care assistants, specialized educators, physiotherapists and speech therapists. It is essential that all these professionals work together, with fluid and continuous communication, to ensure coherent care adapted to the child's evolving needs. The caregiver can play a coordinating role, acting as a link between the family and the various medical and educational services. For example, by taking part in consultation meetings with other professionals, the caregiver can pass on valuable information about the child's condition and the family's needs, while ensuring that care is organized smoothly and efficiently.

**Flexibility in the care plan** is also a fundamental element in working with families. A child's needs may evolve over time, depending on his or her physical, cognitive and emotional development. Similarly, the family situation may change, necessitating adjustments in the organization of care. It is therefore essential that the care plan be flexible enough to adapt to these changes. For example, a child whose health status deteriorates may require intensified medical care or a reorganization of educational support. Conversely, a child who is progressing and becoming more independent may benefit from a reduction in certain assistance arrangements. Working closely with the family, the caregiver can help identify when adjustments are needed, and propose solutions adapted to the child's new needs.

**Emotional support for families** is also an integral part of long-term care planning. Parents of children with disabilities may be faced with feelings of stress, guilt, or worry about their child's future. The caregiver, as a person of trust, can play an emotionally supportive role by listening to parents' concerns and reassuring them that they are not alone in facing these challenges. This can include discussions on the various aspects of the child's disability, but also moments of active listening where parents can share their difficulties and doubts. The caregiver can also refer families to additional resources, such as support groups, parent associations or counseling services, to help them cope with the emotional challenges of long-term care.

**Anticipating life transitions** is another important dimension of long-term care planning. As a child grows, he or she will go through several key stages of development, such as the transition from childhood to adolescence, and then to adulthood. Each of these stages may require adjustments in the care and support provided by family and professionals. For example, the transition to adolescence may involve discussions about puberty, managing autonomy, or planning a more independent life project for the future. It is essential that these transitions are anticipated and prepared for in collaboration with the family, so that the child can benefit from ongoing, tailored support at every stage of life. The caregiver can help identify the key moments when adjustments are needed and guide parents in preparing for these transitions, while ensuring that the child is involved in the process to the best of his or her ability.

**Parent awareness and training** are also essential elements of collaboration in long-term care planning. Although parents may know their child inside out, they may lack the specific skills needed to manage complex medical or educational needs. The caregiver can play an educational role by training parents in certain care gestures, in the use of specific medical equipment, or in adapted communication techniques. For example, for children with motor disorders, the caregiver can teach parents mobilization techniques to avoid injury, or train them in the use of technical aids, such as wheelchairs or transfer devices. This approach enables parents to feel more competent and confident in the day-to-day management of their child's care, while reinforcing their autonomy.

• **Bridging services and support for school leavers**

Relay services and support at the end of the education system play a fundamental role in the transition of young people with disabilities towards an autonomous and fulfilling adult life. This period, marked by the end of schooling, is a key stage that involves many changes - educational, social, professional and personal. For these young people, leaving the often structured and protective school environment can be a source of stress and uncertainty. That's why it's essential to provide them with tailor-made support, adapted to their specific needs, to enable them to access bridging services and benefit from the support they need to be included in society, whether in the field of work, vocational training or social life.

**Support for young people leaving the education system** begins well before the end of their schooling, with early preparation that takes into account their aspirations, abilities and particular needs. The aim is to build a realistic and achievable life project, taking into account the wishes of the young person and his or her family. This may include access to suitable vocational training, integration into a sheltered work environment, or the provision of support to develop the skills needed for independent living. The role of professionals, in particular specialized educators, teachers and care assistants, is to work together to draw up a personalized support project (PPA), which defines the steps to be taken so that the young person can leave the school system with the confidence and resources needed to integrate into society.

**The bridging services that are put** in place at this pivotal moment are essential to ensure a smooth transition. These services, whether medical, educational or social, ensure that young people do not suddenly find themselves without support once they leave the education system. For example, bridging services can include day structures, where young people can take part in activities adapted to their abilities, while continuing to benefit from therapeutic or educational support. These services offer an intermediary framework between school and professional integration, enabling young people to develop social, relational and sometimes even professional skills, while being supervised by trained professionals. They are a place where young people can continue to progress at their own pace, while preparing their transition to greater autonomy.

**Access to vocational training** is one of the mainstays of support after leaving the education system. For many young people with disabilities, adapted vocational training represents a concrete opportunity to acquire skills and integrate into the world of work. Such training is often offered in specialized centers, where programs are adapted to the abilities and pace of the young people concerned. They may include work placements, practical workshops or more theoretical training, depending on the needs and aspirations of each young person. The role of healthcare professionals, and nursing assistants in particular, is to support these young people in this process, ensuring that the training they choose is in line not only with their abilities, but also with their desires. It's crucial that these training courses are not imposed, but that they correspond to the young person's interests, so that they can project themselves into a motivating professional future suited to their talents.

**Support for professional integration** is another key aspect of our support. While some young people can find employment in a mainstream environment, others will need a sheltered work environment, where their disability is taken into account and where they can progress at their own pace. Adapted companies or Etablissements et services d'aide par le travail (ESAT) are specialized structures that offer people with disabilities a professional environment where they can flourish while benefiting from specific support. The caregiver, in collaboration with the other players in the network, can act as an intermediary between the young person and these structures, facilitating his or her integration into the professional environment and ensuring that he or she has the support needed to succeed. This support is all the more important as professional integration can be a determining factor in a young person's self-esteem and place in society.

**Support for social life and independence** is also an integral part of aftercare services. For many young people with disabilities, social life can be a challenge, due to their dependence on a structured environment or difficulties in developing interpersonal relationships. Relay services often offer social and leisure activities that enable young people to continue to develop outside their educational or professional environment. These activities, whether adapted sports, creative workshops or cultural outings, are all opportunities for young people to develop their independence, self-confidence and social skills. By taking part in these activities, they can create a network of relationships and develop interests that help them build a rich and fulfilling social life.

**Managing daily autonomy** is a crucial aspect of this transition. Young people with disabilities may need support to learn how to manage their daily lives more independently, whether in terms of personal hygiene, money management, cooking or getting around.

Bridging services can include programs to teach these basic skills, so that young people can gain independence and feel more empowered in their daily lives. The carer can play a guiding role in this process, teaching the young person practical skills and encouraging them to develop their ability to make decisions for themselves. This can include tasks as simple as running errands or organizing one's schedule, but which, for a young person with a disability, represent important steps towards autonomy.

**The role of families in this transition** is also fundamental. Parents, who are often very involved in their child's school and educational life, may feel a certain anxiety about leaving the education system and entering a new phase in their child's life. It is essential to include them fully in the transition planning process, and to support them in their role as intermediaries. Support for parents can include information sessions on their rights and the assistance available, meetings with professionals, or support groups where they can share their experiences with other families. The caregiver, in conjunction with the other players in the network, can also help them draw up a life project for their child, taking into account both the young person's abilities and the family's wishes.

Finally, **the administrative and legal aspects of** this transition must not be overlooked. Many young people with disabilities benefit from specific rights or social benefits that may change after they leave the education system. Families, who are often faced with complex administrative procedures, need to be informed and supported to ensure that the young person continues to benefit from the necessary assistance. The caregiver can play a mediating role with administrative services, helping to fill out files, understand the young person's rights and access available resources, such as disabled adult allowances (AAH) or independent living aids.

# 11.

# Dealing with behavioral disorders and crisis management

- **Identify triggers for aggressive or self-aggressive behavior**

Identifying the triggers of aggressive or self-aggressive behavior in children or young people with disabilities is a crucial aspect of their care. These behaviors, which are often poorly understood, are frequently manifestations of malaise, frustration or an inability to communicate in any other way. Rather than seeing them as "problem" behaviors, it is essential to understand their root causes and triggers, in order to intervene appropriately and provide the necessary responses. This not only helps prevent their recurrence, but also offers children alternative strategies for expressing their needs and emotions more constructively.

**The first step in identifying triggers** is careful observation of the child and his environment. Aggressive or self-aggressive behaviors never occur without reason: they are often the response to an external or internal stimulus, be it a stressful situation, a change in the environment, physical pain or an unmet need. To understand these behaviors, it's essential to step back and analyze the circumstances that precede them. For example, some children may become aggressive when overwhelmed by sensory stimuli they can't cope with, such as loud noises, bright lights or crowds. Others may react aggressively when they feel frustrated because they can't communicate a need or emotion. Careful observation can help identify these patterns and better understand what triggers the behavior.

**Communication disorders** are frequently at the root of aggressive or self-aggressive behavior, particularly in children with autism spectrum disorders or intellectual disabilities. When a child is unable to express his needs or emotions verbally, he may use aggressive behavior as a means of communicating his frustration or distress. For example, a child who can't express that he's tired, angry or uncomfortable, may hit or shout to express his discomfort. In this case, aggression becomes a means of gaining attention or signalling an unmet need. Identifying triggers in this context requires careful analysis of the situation: what need or emotion is the child trying to communicate? Once the trigger has been identified, alternative communication strategies can be put in place, such as the use of pictograms, sign language or assisted communication devices, to enable the child to express himself in a different way.

**Sensory triggers** are also a frequent cause of aggressive or self-aggressive behavior, particularly in hypersensitive children or those with sensory disorders. Some children can be extremely sensitive to sensory stimuli that others tolerate without difficulty. For example, a sudden noise, an unpleasant texture or unwanted physical contact can trigger an aggressive or withdrawn reaction. It is therefore essential to identify these sensory triggers by carefully observing the child's environment. A room that's too noisy, lighting that's too bright, or uncomfortable clothing, for example, can be the source of agitated or aggressive behavior. The caregiver, in collaboration with parents and educators, can work to modify the child's environment to eliminate or reduce these triggering stimuli. This may include using earmuffs, adapting lighting or suggesting more comfortable clothing.

**Physical pain** is another major trigger for aggressive or self-aggressive behavior. Children who have difficulty verbalizing or expressing their feelings may react to pain by hitting, biting or scratching. It is therefore crucial to consider pain as a possible cause when observing this type of behavior. For example, a child suffering from headaches, dental problems or abdominal pain may manifest his or her discomfort through self-aggressive behaviors, such as head-banging or hand-biting. Observing physical signs, such as grimaces of pain, unusual body postures or unexplained crying, can help identify pain as a trigger. Once pain is suspected, it's essential to consult a healthcare professional to diagnose and treat the underlying cause.

**Stress and anxiety** are also important triggers for aggressive behavior, particularly in situations where the child feels overwhelmed or faced with unexpected change. Some children react to uncertainty or the unknown with aggressive behavior, because they don't know how else to manage their anxiety. For example, a sudden change in routine, such as an unplanned move or a new activity, can generate significant stress in a child who has difficulty adapting to transitions. This stress may manifest itself in aggressive or self-aggressive behavior. In this context, identifying the trigger involves analyzing recent events and changes in the child's routine. Once the trigger has been identified, strategies can be put in place to reduce stress, such as preparing in advance, using visual aids to explain the changes, or introducing moments of relaxation to help the child manage his anxiety.

**Frustration linked to a lack of autonomy** is also a factor that can trigger aggressive or self-aggressive behavior. Children who feel unable to carry out a task, or who are dependent on others to perform simple actions, can feel a deep sense of frustration. This frustration can build up and translate into aggressive behavior when they feel powerless or misunderstood. For example, a child who wants to dress himself but can't may react by getting angry or hitting himself, because he can't express his desire for independence in any other way. In such cases, it is essential to understand that these behaviors reflect a need for autonomy, and to encourage the child to develop skills adapted to his or her level. The caregiver can help the child learn simple gestures by offering progressive support, while rewarding each small success to boost self-confidence.

**The role of social interactions** in triggering aggressive behavior should not be underestimated. Children with disabilities may have difficulty understanding or interpreting social interactions, which can lead to misunderstanding or frustration. For example, a child who feels rejected by his or her peers, or who fails to integrate into a group, may react with aggression or withdrawal. Similarly, a child who doesn't understand the rules of a game, or who feels excluded, may express his frustration by behaving aggressively towards others. In these situations, it's crucial to observe social dynamics and identify moments when the child feels isolated or misunderstood. By encouraging positive social interactions and teaching communication and conflict management skills, these behaviors can be prevented.




- **De-escalation techniques and crisis management**

De-escalation techniques and crisis management are essential strategies for supporting children with disabilities, especially those who are likely to display aggressive or self-aggressive behaviors at times of great emotional turmoil. These behaviors may be the result of frustration, anxiety, pain or an inability to communicate in any other way. At such times, it's crucial to intervene in a calm and controlled manner in order to de-escalate the situation, protect the child and those around him/her, and prevent the crisis from escalating. De-escalation involves gradually reducing the intensity of the situation, calming the child and helping him or her to return to a more stable emotional state. To achieve this, caregivers and other support professionals need to master specific techniques and adopt a caring, patient and empathetic attitude.

**The first step in de-escalation** is to **remain calm** and manage your own emotions. In the face of a crisis, it's natural to feel stressed or worried, but it's essential for the caregiver to remain calm, as his or her attitude and behavior directly influence the child's state. If the adult responds to agitation with anger or panic, the situation is likely to get worse. On the other hand, calm, collected behavior can help defuse tension. Speaking softly, in simple, clear sentences, without raising your voice, helps to create a calming environment. Tone of voice, body language and facial expression are crucial in showing the child that the adult remains in control of the situation and is there to help, not to reprimand or control.

**Active listening** is another key technique for de-escalating crises. It involves showing the child that his feelings are understood and heard, even if he is unable to express them verbally. By listening attentively and rephrasing what we perceive to be his emotional state, we can help him put words to his emotions and feel validated in what he's going through. For example, when faced with an angry or crying child, saying "I can see that you're very angry, that something's bothering you" can help them feel understood, which is often the first step towards appeasement. This kind of rephrasing helps reduce the feeling of injustice or misunderstanding that can exacerbate the crisis. The child feels that the adult is not judging him or her, but trying to understand and help him or her through this difficult time.

**Physical space management** is also important in de-escalation. If the child is in an environment where he feels overwhelmed by sensory stimuli, such as loud noises or crowds, it can be helpful to move him to a quieter, less stimulating place. Sometimes, offering the child a safe space, free from distractions and threats, can reduce the pressure he feels and help him relax. This can be a quiet room, a quiet corner with familiar objects, or even an outdoor area. The aim is to create a space where the child can regain a sense of security and is less exposed to stress or frustration triggers.

**Distraction techniques** are often effective in diverting a child's attention from a stressful or frustrating event. The idea is to offer an activity or object that draws the child's attention away from the source of the crisis. This could be a simple game, a sensory object, a drawing or an activity that the child particularly enjoys. For example, for a child who is beginning to show signs of agitation, suggesting that they look together at an illustrated book or handle a stress ball may be enough to divert their mind from the cause of their frustration. This technique works well with children who have difficulty managing strong emotions and need to focus on something positive to calm them down.

**Non-verbal communication** also plays a crucial role in crisis management. Sometimes, children in crisis are too overwhelmed by their emotions to process verbal information. The caregiver can then use gentle gestures, open postures and reassuring proximity to communicate a sense of security. For example, sitting at the childs' level, avoiding abrupt gestures and maintaining a respectful distance are ways of showing the child that the adult is there to help without invading. These non-verbal gestures of support can be enough to calm a tense situation, showing the child that he or she is safe and doesn't have to defend or oppose.

**The importance of routine** in crisis management should not be underestimated. Children, particularly those with autism spectrum disorders or intellectual disabilities, often react badly to unexpected changes or a lack of reference points. Establishing structured routines reduces uncertainty and reassures the child about what's going to happen next. When the child is faced with an unexpected change or situation, the caregiver can use a visual aid (such as an illustrated schedule) to explain what's going to happen and reassure the child that the situation is under control. This helps limit anxiety-related crises and feelings of loss of control. For example, before a doctor's appointment or a trip, you can show the child the stages of what's going to happen, so that he or she feels prepared and less stressed.

**The technique of positive reinforcement** can be very useful in managing tantrums and preventing their recurrence. It involves recognizing and rewarding the child's calm, positive behavior, even in situations where the child is calming down after a crisis. For example, if the child starts to calm down again after a phase of agitation, the caregiver can congratulate him on his efforts by saying: "Bravo, you've managed to calm down, that's very good." This approach enables the child to understand that his efforts to manage his emotions are recognized and encouraged, which reinforces the desire to reproduce these behaviors in future situations.

Finally, **crisis management must always be accompanied by retrospective evaluation**. Once the situation has calmed down, it's important to step back and reflect on what triggered the crisis, what worked to de-escalate it, and what could be improved in the future. This analysis enables us to better anticipate crises and implement preventive strategies. Together, professionals and parents can think about ways to prevent these situations from arising in the first place, by identifying the specific triggers for each child. This retrospective reflection also enables us to better understand the child, his or her needs and communication patterns, and to provide more personalized support.

- **Apply methods such as *Positive Behaviour Support (PBS)***

Applying methods such as **Positive Behaviour Support (PBS)** is a structured, caring approach to managing challenging behaviours in people with disabilities. This framework is based on a thorough understanding of the underlying reasons for challenging behaviors, and aims to improve the individual's quality of life by promoting adaptive and socially acceptable behaviors. PBS does not focus solely on reducing undesirable behaviors, but seeks above all to promote positive behaviors and strengthen the individual's social, emotional and behavioral skills, taking into account his or her environment and specific needs.

## Understanding Positive Behaviour Support (PBS)

PBS is based on the idea that **all behavior has a function**, whether it's a way for the individual to communicate a need, express frustration or react to a stressful situation. For example, a child who starts shouting or hitting could be doing so because he's overwhelmed by sensory stimuli, frustrated at not being able to express himself, or seeking to avoid a task he finds difficult. PBS therefore focuses on identifying the **root causes** of problem behaviors, so that strategies can be put in place to avoid them and replace them with more appropriate behaviors.

**PBS pillars include:**

1. **Functional analysis of behavior**: This involves understanding why a behavior occurs by analyzing the events that precede it (antecedents) and the consequences

that reinforce it. The aim is to identify the specific triggers (stimuli, context) and environmental responses that maintain the behavior.

2.  **Proactive intervention**: Instead of waiting for the undesirable behavior to manifest itself, PBS aims to **modify the environment** to avoid the situations that trigger these behaviors. This can include setting up structured routines, adapting activities, reducing sensory stimuli, or anticipating moments of stress.

3.  **Positive behavior reinforcement**: PBS focuses on **learning new behaviors**, by positively reinforcing desired actions. This means that every time a child or person adopts a positive behavior, it should be rewarded with some form of reinforcement: it could be verbal praise, a smile, or an activity enjoyed. This positive reinforcement helps create a link between adapted behaviors and pleasant consequences, making these behaviors more likely to recur.

4.  **Interventions tailored to individual needs**: Every PBS plan is individualized. What works for one person may not work for another. The approach is therefore personalized, taking into account the **abilities**, **preferences** and specific **difficulties** of each individual.

## The steps involved in setting up a PBS

### 1. Functional behavior analysis

The first step in PBS is to carry out a **Functional Behavioral Assessment** (FBA). This assessment is based on careful observation of the person in different situations, to understand why he or she adopts certain behaviors. It's essential to ask the question: **"What is the purpose of this behavior for this person?"** For example, a child may display aggression to gain attention, avoid a difficult task, or escape sensory overload. Analysis helps determine what the person is trying to communicate through their behavior, which then becomes the basis for intervention.

## 2. Prevention and environmental modification

Having identified the underlying causes of the behavior, the next step is to **adapt the** environment **to** eliminate or minimize the triggers. If a child reacts aggressively when overwhelmed by loud noises, it may be helpful to offer a quiet space where he can retreat when it becomes too much to handle. If frustration arises from communication difficulties, the use of alternative communication tools, such as pictograms or Makaton, can reduce problem behaviors. **Anticipating needs** and breaking points can help defuse situations before they reach a critical point.

## 3. Teaching new skills

PBS places a strong emphasis on **teaching behavioral alternatives**. The idea is to help the person learn more acceptable and effective ways of meeting their needs. For example, a child who starts shouting for attention can be encouraged to ask for help verbally or to raise his or her hand in a school setting. This learning process may take time, but it relies on a caring and patient approach, with regular repetition and constant positive reinforcement.

## 4. Positive reinforcement

Positive reinforcement is central to PBS. When the child or person adopts a more appropriate behavior, it's essential to **reward** this behavior **immediately** to create a clear link between the positive action and the reward. This reinforcement can take many forms: verbal praise, favorite activities, or simply positive attention. The aim is to create positive experiences around the desired behaviors so that they become more frequent. Ultimately, this helps to reduce undesirable behaviors by replacing them with adapted behaviors that bring similar benefits to the individual.

## 5. Monitoring and adjusting the plan

The PBS is not a fixed approach; it requires constant monitoring and regular adjustments. Behaviors evolve, and the plan must evolve with them. So it's important to **monitor progress**, review what's working and what's not, and modify the plan accordingly. For example, if a certain positive behavior emerges, but other undesirable behaviors persist, it may be necessary to examine new environmental or social factors influencing these behaviors.

## The benefits of Positive Behaviour Support

**1. Improved quality of life**: By focusing on prevention, education and positive reinforcement, PBS can significantly improve the quality of life of the people it supports. Not only do undesirable behaviors diminish, but the person also develops new skills, greater self-esteem and greater autonomy.

**2. Reducing problem behaviors**: One of the strengths of PBS is its ability to reduce undesirable behaviors without resorting to sanctions or punishment. By understanding the function of the behavior and providing alternative solutions, the approach enables these behaviors to be progressively reduced, while offering responses that are better adapted to the person's needs.

**3. Individualized, caring approach**: PBS respects each person's individuality and adopts a caring approach, centered on his or her needs and environment. By reinforcing positive behaviors, this method promotes a relational dynamic based on respect and encouragement, while offering concrete tools for overcoming behavioral difficulties.

- **Preventing crisis situations through observation and proactive prevention**

Preventing crisis situations in children and young people with disabilities is a fundamental issue in their support. Rather than waiting for crises to erupt and then reacting, it is preferable to adopt a proactive approach based on careful observation and prevention. This approach not only helps prevent crises from occurring, but also creates a more serene environment, adapted to the specific needs of each child. By being attentive to early warning signs and intervening before the situation degenerates, we can help the child better manage his or her emotions and avoid aggressive or self-aggressive behavior.

## Observation as the key to prevention

Careful, ongoing observation of the child is the essential first step in preventing seizures. Every child is unique, and it's important to understand the **warning signs** or **subtle clues** that indicate a seizure is about to occur. These signs can be anything from physical agitation, to a change in tone of voice, withdrawal, muscle tension or a change in general attitude. For example, a child who starts rubbing his face or avoiding eye contact could be signalling that he's feeling overwhelmed by a stressful situation. Identifying these signs allows you to react quickly and defuse the situation before it escalates.

Observation should not be limited to the child himself, but should encompass his **immediate environment**. It is important to take into account the context in which the child evolves: the people present, the noise level, the complexity of the tasks required, or even the structure of the day. For example, a child may be more likely to face a crisis in a noisy environment, or after a day without a break. By observing these external elements, it becomes easier to identify recurring **triggers** and act accordingly.

## Preventing crises with a structured routine

One of the most effective ways of preventing crises is to establish a **structured, predictable routine**. Children with disabilities, especially those with autism spectrum disorders or communication difficulties, can be very sensitive to change or the unexpected. A well-established routine enables them to know in advance what's going to happen, to prepare mentally for transitions, and to feel secure in a familiar environment. This structure reduces anxiety linked to uncertainty and helps them to manage transitions better.

The use of **visual aids** or **illustrated schedules** is particularly beneficial in helping children anticipate the day's events. For example, pictograms representing different activities (such as breakfast, school or playtime) can be arranged in a precise order to give the child an overview of what to expect. This allows the child to prepare for each stage, reducing the risk of unpleasant surprises that could trigger a crisis.

## Adapting the environment to minimize triggers

The link between the environment and a child's behavior is often very strong. Certain **sensory stimuli** can trigger emotional overload, especially in hypersensitive children. This can be due to loud noises, bright lights, uncomfortable textures or uncontrolled social interactions. It is therefore essential to **create a calm environment adapted to the** child's specific sensory needs.

For example, for a child who is sensitive to noise, it may be useful to provide **noise-cancelling headphones** or quiet areas where he can retreat to in case of sensory overload. Similarly, room lighting can be adjusted, avoiding overly bright or flashing lights that can aggravate stress. The layout of the room should also be designed to reduce excessive stimulation: soothing colors, familiar objects or isolated corners can help to calm the child and prevent seizures.

## Encourage communication to avoid frustration

Crises are often the result of frustration linked to a child's inability to express his needs or emotions. To prevent these situations, it is essential to **develop alternative means of**

**communication** that enable the child to express himself more easily. The use of **pictograms**, **sign language** (such as Makaton), or **communication tablets** can help the child indicate clearly what he or she needs, whether it's a break, help with a difficult task, or simply attention.

Adults also need to **adapt their communication** to the child, using simple sentences, giving him enough time to respond, and making sure he understands what is being asked of him. A child who doesn't understand what's expected of him can quickly become stressed or frustrated, which can lead to a crisis. By being clear and giving instructions adapted to their abilities, we reduce confusion and therefore the risk of difficult behavior.

## Positive reinforcement and encouragement of appropriate behavior

A proactive crisis prevention strategy also involves **positive reinforcement** of appropriate behaviors. Rather than focusing solely on the moments when a child displays difficult behaviors, it's important to value every effort and every positive behavior. When a child uses emotional regulation strategies or expresses his needs in an adapted way, it's crucial to praise him or offer him a reward. This shows him that his positive behaviors are recognized and encouraged, and that he is able to manage his emotions in a constructive way.

For example, if a child starts to show signs of agitation but manages to calm down using a learned technique (such as deep breathing or handling a soothing object), it's essential to recognize this effort and reinforce it with verbal encouragement or a tangible reward (such as extra time for an activity he or she enjoys). This type of reinforcement encourages the child to reproduce these behaviors in future situations, helping to prevent the onset of seizures.

# Proactive intervention and transition management

**Transitions** are often delicate moments for children, especially those with autism spectrum disorders or emotional regulation difficulties. Moving from one activity to another, leaving a familiar place or preparing for an unexpected event can provoke heightened anxiety. To prevent these transitions from triggering a crisis, it's helpful to **prepare the child in advance** by explaining what's going to happen and giving him or her time cues.

Using **visual countdowns** or **stopwatches** helps to anticipate the end of one activity and the start of another. For example, before changing activities, you can say to the child: "In five minutes, we're going to put the toys away and move on to reading", by showing him an hourglass or stopwatch. This reduces the anxiety associated with sudden transitions and gives the child time to adjust to the idea of change. What's more, clearly announcing what's going to happen next gives the child a sense of control and security.

# Encouraging autonomy and involvement

Finally, it's important to **encourage the** child's **autonomy** by allowing him to make choices and participate actively in his daily activities. Crises can sometimes occur when children feel powerless or constrained in their actions. By offering developmentally appropriate choices, children are given the opportunity to take part in decision-making and have some control over their environment. This can be as simple as allowing him to choose between two activities, to decide on the order of tasks, or to choose a break whenever he wants. This proactive approach boosts the child's self-confidence and reduces feelings of frustration or helplessness, which can often be at the root of tantrums.

# 12.

# Palliative and end-of-life care for children with disabilities

- **Understanding the specificity of palliative care for disabled children**

Palliative care for children with disabilities is a specific and delicate field, requiring a deep understanding of each child's particular needs, as well as the emotional impact on the family. Unlike palliative care for adults, which often focuses on terminal illness at the end of life, pediatric palliative care can extend over long periods, sometimes several years. It aims to improve the child's quality of life by managing pain and symptoms and providing holistic support tailored to his or her physical, emotional and psychosocial needs. In the case of children with disabilities, this approach is even more complex, since we have to take into account their overall state of health, their capacities and the specificities linked to their disability, while accompanying them in their development despite their illness.

## A holistic, individualized approach to palliative care

Palliative care for disabled children requires a **holistic approach**, i.e. it must consider the child as a whole, taking into account not only the physical aspects of the illness, but also the emotional, social and spiritual dimensions. This means adapting interventions to both the symptoms of the disease and the needs associated with the disability. Each child is unique, and so must be his or her care. Care teams must therefore build an individualized care plan that takes into account not only the child's medical condition, but also his or her ability to communicate, move, interact with the environment and express comfort or discomfort.

For example, a child with severe cerebral palsy who cannot speak will have difficulty expressing pain or emotions. In this context, it is essential to use specific pain assessment tools, such as facial expressions or behavioral changes, to adapt treatment appropriately. In addition, these children may have complex health problems requiring ongoing medical care, such as respiratory disorders or feeding difficulties, which need to be taken into account in the overall management of their comfort and well-being.

## Pain and symptom management

One of the main aims of palliative care is to **relieve the pain and uncomfortable symptoms** a child may be experiencing. In children with disabilities, this can be more complex due to communication difficulties or multiple associated pathologies. It is therefore crucial to adapt pain assessments to the child's ability to express himself. Caregivers need to be alert to subtle signs such as changes in behavior, unusual body movements, moaning or altered eating habits, which may indicate pain or discomfort.

Symptom management also requires a multidisciplinary approach, involving doctors, nurses, physiotherapists, care assistants, psychologists and social workers. Together, they assess the child's needs and implement strategies to improve comfort. For example, for a child with respiratory problems, the care team may use respiratory physiotherapy techniques or specific equipment to facilitate breathing and reduce distress. Nutrition, managing recurrent infections and preventing bedsores are also key elements of palliative care for children with severe physical disabilities.

## Supporting children's development despite illness

One of the specific challenges of pediatric palliative care **is to continue to support the child's development**, even when the illness is incurable. Unlike adults, children continue to grow, learn and develop, even when receiving palliative care. It is therefore essential to provide them with a stimulating environment that supports their personal development, while managing the symptoms of the disease. This can include activities adapted to their abilities, such as sensory play, socializing with other children or learning sessions tailored to their cognitive needs.

The aim of palliative care for these children is not simply to prolong life, but to **improve its quality**, enabling the child to live life to the fullest, to the best of his or her abilities, while being surrounded by a caring environment. This approach requires close communication with parents to determine care objectives, based on the family's wishes and expectations. For example, some parents may want their child to continue attending school for as long as possible, even if this means specific adaptations and increased support, while others may prefer a quieter environment at home.

## The central role of families in palliative care

Palliative care concerns not only the child, but also his or her family, who play a central role in day-to-day support. Parents of disabled children are often heavily involved in their child's care, and can feel helpless as the disease progresses. They have to deal with the day-to-day management of care, the pain of seeing their child suffer, and the prospect of a potentially fatal outcome. It is therefore crucial to offer them **emotional and psychological support**, while actively involving them in care decisions.

Palliative care teams need to work hand-in-hand with families to understand their wishes, fears and priorities. **Open communication** is essential to help parents anticipate and prepare for the various stages of the illness, while respecting their choices. For example, some families may prefer home care to offer their child a more familiar and warm environment, while others may prefer specialized services such as pediatric palliative care units, which offer more intensive medical supervision.

Support for siblings is also an often overlooked but crucial aspect of palliative care. The siblings of a seriously ill child may experience anxiety, jealousy or a feeling of being left out because of the attention paid to the sick child. So it's important to include them in the process, explain the situation in an age-appropriate way, and offer them space to express their own emotions.

# Psychological support and spiritual care

In palliative care, **psychological support** and **spiritual care** take on particular importance. For children, living with an incurable illness can generate anxiety, sadness or fear. It is therefore essential to offer them a safe space in which to express their emotions, whether through speech, play or creative activities. Health professionals, whether psychologists, educators or care assistants, must be attentive to the child's emotional needs, adapting their approach according to the child's age, cognitive abilities and level of understanding of the situation.

**Spiritual care** can also be important for some children and their families, depending on their religious beliefs or their need to find meaning in illness. Whether through religious rituals, discussions about death or moments of reflection, this care aims to provide comfort, ease end-of-life anxieties and offer moral support.

# Anticipating transitions and end-of-life phases

Finally, a difficult but inescapable aspect of palliative care for children with disabilities is **preparation for the end of life**. For many families, accepting this reality is a complex emotional process. Professionals must accompany families through this stage, helping them to anticipate critical phases, while offering them tools to get through this period with dignity and serenity. Decisions about end-of-life care, such as the use of pain-relieving treatments or the decision to stop certain invasive treatments, must be taken in consultation with the family, respecting their values and their vision of their child's comfort.

- **Helping families through difficult times: psychological support**

Accompanying families through difficult times, particularly when faced with the illness, disability or end of life of a child, is a delicate and essential mission for caregivers. **Psychological support** plays a central role in this process, enabling parents, siblings and loved ones to get through these difficult times with solid emotional and moral support. When a child's health is at stake, the whole family is often plunged into a turmoil of complex emotions: fear, sadness, anger, guilt and helplessness. The role of caregivers, in particular orderlies, psychologists and nurses, is to be present to listen, understand, soothe and offer resources adapted to each stage of the child's illness or disability.

## The importance of listening with empathy and kindness

**Psychological support** for families begins with **empathetic listening** and constant availability. Parents of a sick or disabled child often experience intense stress, which can sometimes be exacerbated by uncertainty about the course of the illness or disability. It is therefore essential that caregivers listen to their concerns, fears and questions, without judgement or haste. This active listening creates a bond of trust with families, who need to feel understood and supported in the darkest moments.

Empathetic listening is not simply about gathering information, but about **providing a space where** parents can express their feelings, even those that are difficult to articulate, such as anger or despair. Sometimes, parents feel guilty for feeling angry or helpless about their child's situation, and need reassurance that these emotions are natural. As caregivers, it's important to validate these emotions, offer them a safe space to express them, and help them navigate through this emotional complexity.

## Understanding and coping with the shock of diagnosis

When a diagnosis of disability or serious illness is made, the family is often faced with an intense emotional shock. **The announcement of a diagnosis** such as a physical handicap or progressive illness triggers a strong emotional reaction, often combining denial, sadness, anger and fear of the future. For parents, it's a moment when the dream of a "normal" life for their child collapses, giving way to many questions and anxieties.

The role of the caregivers **at** this stage is to **support the family in accepting the diagnosis**, and to accompany them in this process of mourning, not for the child itself, but for the life project they had for it. This often requires a gentle presence, an ability to welcome complex emotions and, above all, not to rush parents through this stage. Everyone has their own pace when it comes to accepting such a reality, and it's important to respect this rhythm while offering regular, appropriate support.

Caregivers must also ensure that they offer clear, comprehensible information about the child's situation. Faced with the shock of a diagnosis, it's easy for parents to feel overwhelmed by medical terms or prognoses. Caregivers can play a mediating role by explaining in a simple, human way what the diagnosis entails, while answering questions in a calming manner. Sometimes, simply understanding what's going on can help alleviate some of the anguish and begin the process of acceptance.

## Supporting the family throughout the treatment process

Beyond the initial shock, **psychological support** must be ongoing throughout the treatment process. A child's illness or disability is often experienced as a long-term ordeal, marked by ups and downs, moments of hope followed by periods of discouragement. Caregivers need to be present at every stage, adapting their support to the emotional needs of the family.

This includes **preparing parents for the different phases of** illness or disability, offering them information about what to expect, and listening to their concerns. Anticipating future difficulties can help them prepare better psychologically, and feel less helpless when complications arise.

Another crucial aspect is to **support parents in managing the complex emotions** that can arise over time. Faced with a chronic illness or progressive disability, psychological fatigue can build up, hopes can be dashed, and conflicts can emerge within the family. Caregivers, and psychologists in particular, can offer tools to manage stress, develop relaxation techniques, and provide forums for unloading accumulated tensions.

## Supporting siblings

When providing psychological support to families, it's essential not to forget the **siblings** of a sick or disabled child. They may experience contradictory emotions, ranging from concern for their brother or sister to feelings of jealousy or frustration at the increased attention the sick child receives. It's important to create moments when siblings can express their own emotions and feel listened to. They need to understand the situation in an age-appropriate way, and be reassured of their own place in the family.

Caregivers can also help parents manage this **complex family dynamic**, offering advice on how to include siblings in the care process, while ensuring that they don't feel neglected. Organizing special times for them, when they can have their parents' undivided attention, can help balance family relationships and reduce tensions.

## Support at the end of life: intensified support

When a child is terminally ill, **psychological support** takes on an even more intense and delicate dimension. This period is often marked by deep emotional pain, for parents and relatives alike. The role of caregivers here is to provide ongoing emotional support, helping parents cope with this difficult reality and make decisions that respect their values and wishes for their child's end-of-life.

At such times, it's essential to **offer a safe space for the** most painful **emotions**. Parents may feel guilt, anger or even relief at the imminent end of their child's suffering. These emotions, though difficult to experience, are natural and should be welcomed without judgment. Caregivers need to create a framework in which these feelings can be expressed, while providing a comforting presence.

End-of-life support also includes managing **mourning rituals**. For some parents, preparation for their child's end-of-life may include discussions about the funeral, the memories to be created or specific moments of farewell. Caregivers can guide them through this process, respecting their spiritual or religious beliefs and needs. Support doesn't stop with the death of the child: parents need ongoing support in the weeks and months that follow, to help them get through the bereavement in a caring and accompanied way.

- **Adapting end-of-life care: comfort, dignity and respect for the child**

Adapting end-of-life care for a disabled child is a sensitive process, requiring meticulous attention to every aspect of the child's well-being. The objectives at this stage are to ensure the child's **comfort**, preserve his or her **dignity**, and guarantee **respect for** the person, physically, emotionally and spiritually. The approach to palliative care for children is fundamentally different from that for adults. It is not limited to alleviating physical symptoms, but also includes holistic support, focusing on the particular needs of the child and his or her family, while respecting the child's individuality and life path.

## Ensuring the child's comfort

**Comfort** is the first priority in end-of-life care. This means minimizing, as far as possible, the pain and physical symptoms that accompany the progression of the disease. **Pain management** is essential at this stage. Caregivers must be proactive and anticipate pain by regularly adjusting treatments, whether these involve analgesic drugs such as opioids, or other symptomatic treatments aimed at reducing physical suffering (antinauseants, treatment of dyspnea, etc.). In paediatric care, caregivers need to be particularly attentive to these adjustments, as children cannot always express their pain or discomfort clearly. Careful observation of body signals (changes in posture, facial expressions) is therefore essential.

In addition to medical pain management, the child's **physical comfort** can be ensured by regular, gentle care: light massages, adjustment of position to prevent bedsores, and hygiene care that brings relief and dignity. It's also crucial to create an environment conducive to calm and comfort: the care space must be soothing, whether in hospital or at home. Dimmed lights, familiar objects such as toys, blankets or soft music can contribute to a serene environment, reducing the child's anxiety.

**The family environment** also plays a central role in the comfort of the dying child. For many families, the idea of spending the last days at home, surrounded by loved ones, can offer a more reassuring and welcoming setting than hospital. It also allows a more familiar routine to be maintained, while integrating the necessary medical care. Respecting the child's and family's wishes regarding where care should take place contributes greatly to their overall well-being.

## Preserving the child's dignity

A child's **dignity** must be preserved throughout end-of-life care. This begins with a profound respect for their body and individuality, even when they can no longer clearly express their wishes. Hygiene care, such as washing or changing clothes, must be carried out gently and discreetly, with total respect for the child's modesty and privacy. This care, although simple, is a time to show the child that he or she is cared for with attention and respect, and that every gesture counts.

Preserving the child's dignity also means **respecting his or her choices**, as far as possible. If the child is old enough to understand his or her situation, it is essential to include him or her in decisions concerning his or her care, taking into account the child's ability to express his or her wishes. Some children, even at the end of life, have specific wishes: they may want to spend time with their loved ones, listen to their favorite music or take part in activities that are important to them, even if their state of health no longer allows them to do so intensively. The role of caregivers is to listen to these wishes and respect them as much as possible, so that the child can live these moments with the feeling of being in control of his or her life right up to the end.

Dignity is also reflected in the way the care team and family approach **communication with the child**. It's important to talk sincerely, taking into account the child's age and ability to understand what he's going through. Lying or concealing the reality of his situation can further upset him. So it's essential to establish a caring dialogue, in which the child feels respected for his emotions and fears, without overwhelming him with information he can't handle.

## Respecting individuality and emotional needs

Respecting children at the end of life also means taking into account their **emotional and psychological needs**. Even in their final days, children are still developing beings, with complex emotions that they may not always be able to express. It is therefore essential to be attentive to their emotional needs and the way they perceive their environment. The presence of close relatives, parents and siblings, and the opportunity for the child to maintain strong emotional ties, is fundamental. These moments of sharing, of listening, and sometimes simply of shared silence, enable the child to feel surrounded and loved.

For some children, **spiritual care** can also bring profound relief. This depends on the family's religious or spiritual beliefs, but some children find comfort in prayers, rituals or simply in discussing life and death. Caregivers need to be sensitive to these dimensions and, with the family's agreement, offer appropriate spiritual accompaniment, whether through chapels, religious celebrants or more philosophical discussions.

## Supporting the family at this stage

As well as caring for the child, it's crucial to **support the family** through this difficult time. Parents and relatives are often devastated by the thought of losing their child, and need constant emotional and psychological support. Psychological support must be omnipresent, whether in the form of individual interviews with a psychologist, group sessions for family members, or simply a sympathetic ear from caregivers.

Parents need to be guided through the decision-making process regarding end-of-life care, while being supported in their choices, whatever they may be. Some decisions, such as stopping certain treatments or introducing palliative care only, can be extremely difficult to make. Caregivers must be present to clearly explain the implications of each decision, while respecting the family's values and wishes.

- **Working closely with palliative care teams**

Working closely with palliative care teams is essential to ensure comprehensive and appropriate care for children at the end of life. This collaborative work relies on fluid communication between different healthcare professionals, coordinated actions and a multidisciplinary approach focused on the child's well-being and family support. Palliative care is complex, because it involves not only physical pain management, but also psychological, emotional, social and spiritual dimensions. This complexity makes it essential for doctors, nurses, care assistants, psychologists, social workers and spiritual care specialists to work together to meet all the needs of the child and his or her family.

## Communication: a central element of collaboration

**Communication** between members of the palliative care team is one of the keys to successful collaboration. The professionals involved in the child's care must regularly exchange information on the evolution of the child's state of health, the symptoms he or she presents, and the necessary adjustments to care. These exchanges must be continuous and transparent, so that each professional has a clear view of the situation and can intervene in a coherent, coordinated way.

Multi-disciplinary meetings, where all team members meet to discuss the child's case, are an effective way of ensuring fluid communication. They enable us to pool the observations of the various professionals, adjust treatments according to current needs, and anticipate future steps. At these meetings, each member of the team can share his or her concerns and suggestions, thus enriching overall care. The caregiver, who is in direct contact with the child on a daily basis, plays a central role in these meetings, providing precise information on the child's physical and emotional state, reactions to care and immediate needs.

**The exchange of information** must also be clear and respectful, with particular attention paid to the sensitivity of the subject. It is essential that everyone knows when and how to intervene, whether to adjust a treatment, soothe a pain, or offer emotional support. The aim is to guarantee continuity of care, where each action is part of an overall logic of well-being for the child.

## A multidisciplinary approach to comprehensive care

The **multidisciplinary** approach of palliative care enables us to address the different dimensions of a child's suffering at the end of life, taking into account not only his physical pain, but also his psychological and social needs. Each member of the team brings a specific expertise, but it is the combination of these skills that enables us to meet the complex needs of the child and his or her family.

Doctors, in collaboration with nurses and care assistants, are responsible for **managing physical symptoms** and medical treatments. The role of nurses and orderlies is fundamental, as they are in direct contact with the child and his or her parents, enabling them to adjust care reactively as the child's state of health evolves. The nurse, for example, can adjust the infusion to relieve pain, while the caregiver, through his or her continuous presence, observes subtle signs of comfort or discomfort, and adjusts care accordingly, whether in terms of hygiene, positioning or symptom monitoring.

At the same time, **psychologists** and **social workers** provide emotional support for the child and his or her family. They help parents to understand the situation, to cope with the anticipated bereavement, and to prepare for the end of their child's life in a peaceful way. Psychologists, in particular, are essential in helping children to express their emotions and fears in the face of illness, while creating a safe space where they can verbalize or communicate their emotional needs. They also work closely with caregivers to ensure that the child is surrounded by constant emotional support.

**Spiritual care**, which can be provided by chaplains or spiritual advisors, plays a crucial role for some families, particularly when questions about the meaning of life and death arise. Their interventions help to meet the spiritual needs of the child and those close to him/her, whether religious or more personal, while respecting the beliefs and values of each family. The dialogue between caregivers and spiritual professionals must be open, so that everyone knows when it's appropriate to call on these resources.

## Coordinating care and anticipating needs

Another key aspect of working with palliative care teams is **coordinating care**. It is essential to ensure that all interventions are coordinated and planned according to the progression of the disease. Each member of the team needs to know his or her specific role and how it fits into the child's overall care plan.

One of the major challenges is **to anticipate the** child's **needs**. By working together, professionals can anticipate critical moments, such as a deteriorating state of health or upcoming pain management. Anticipation makes it possible to avoid crises and react quickly when the child shows signs of distress, whether physical or emotional. For example, by anticipating medication adjustments or planning regular psychological support, the team can provide a proactive, rather than reactive, response.

**The flexibility** of this coordination is also crucial. A child's needs can evolve very rapidly, particularly at the end of life, and it's important that the team can adjust its actions in line with these changes. If a symptom worsens or pain appears, caregivers must be able to react quickly, adapting treatment or implementing new interventions to relieve the child.

## Supporting the family in the decision-making process

Medical decisions in palliative care are often complex and delicate. Families are faced with difficult choices, such as whether to stop certain treatments, or whether to prioritize their child's comfort over prolonging life at all costs. The role of caregivers is to **support parents** in these decisions by providing clear, objective information and emotional support.

Collaboration between the various members of the palliative care team enables us to provide **comprehensive support** for parents. Doctors explain the care options available, while psychologists and social workers provide support in navigating the ethical and emotional dilemmas associated with these decisions. It's vital that parents never feel alone when faced with these choices, and that they know they can count on the team to guide them with kindness.

- **The importance of bereavement and supporting families after death**

**Grief** is a deeply personal and unique experience, which occurs after the loss of a loved one. When it involves a child, the grieving process is particularly difficult and can leave families in immense emotional distress. Supporting families after the death of a child with a disability or serious illness is crucial, as it enables them to cope with this difficult stage in their lives, when grief, incomprehension and sometimes guilt can take on considerable importance. Caregivers, especially those who have accompanied the child and family throughout the illness, play an essential role in this support. They must be there to offer comfort, resources and a sympathetic ear, to help the family get through this difficult period and find ways to live with their grief.

## Understanding the importance of grief

Mourning is a natural and necessary process for **coping with loss**. It's not a matter of "turning the page", but of finding a way to integrate this loss into the lives of survivors, to give it meaning and to reorganize one's existence in light of this absence. For parents who have lost a child, this process is often extremely long and complex. The death of a child is an ordeal that many parents describe as unnatural, because it breaks the usual order of life, where it is the parents who are supposed to leave before their children.

**Supporting families after a death** is therefore essential to enable them to express their grief, share their emotions, and not feel alone in this ordeal. It's important to make them understand that grieving is a process unique to each person, that there is no "right" or "wrong" way to grieve, and that each parent, sibling and family member will go through this period at his or her own pace. Some parents may need to talk regularly about their child, sharing memories, while others will need silence, distance or solitude. The aim of our support is to respect this rhythm, to support the family in their choices, and to help them find the resources to get through this period without sinking into destructive grief.

## Offer emotional and psychological support

After the death of a child, families can experience **an immense sense of emptiness**, often mixed with sadness, shock, and sometimes guilt or anger. Psychological support at this time is essential to help them express their emotions and find a space where these feelings can be shared without judgment. The psychologists, social workers and carers who have accompanied them can play an important role in this support, offering them individual interviews or group sessions.

It's also essential to encourage parents **not to repress their emotions**, even when they seem too painful to express. Some families may find it difficult to talk about their child's death, for fear of reopening wounds or upsetting those around them. Yet expressing grief, whether through words, rituals or symbolic activities, is an important way of giving meaning to the loss and moving forward in the grieving process.

**The** deceased child's **siblings**, who are often forgotten in this dynamic, must also be included in this support. They may feel confused, guilty or even jealous of the attention the sick child received before death. Caregivers need to ensure that they have the space to express themselves, through therapeutic games, age-appropriate discussions, or even bereavement groups. This helps them to understand and deal with their own grief, while preventing them from feeling marginalized or abandoned at this time.

## Supporting the family in the aftermath of death

After the death of a child, parents are often overwhelmed by a **whirlwind of administrative and practical** procedures, which they must manage despite their grief. Caregivers can also play an invaluable role here. Helping families to organize their child's **funeral**, understand the legal procedures associated with the death, and deal with administrative issues enables them to concentrate on their grief and alleviate some of the logistical burden.

Funerals are a key moment in the grieving process, marking a symbolic step in the acceptance of loss. Caregivers can help parents reflect on how they wish to organize this event: choosing a ritual that reflects the family's values, creating moments to share memories of the child, or personalizing the funeral with elements that were dear to him or her. These gestures give meaning to this stage of the process, and honor the child's memory in a way that respects both the parents' grief and their child's uniqueness.

## The role of long-term follow-up

Supporting families doesn't have to stop at the funeral. **Long-term follow-up** is just as important, because mourning is a process that lasts well beyond the first few weeks after death. Many parents feel a form of isolation after the funeral, when the attention of loved ones begins to dissipate and the reality of the child's absence settles into everyday life. Caregivers can help maintain a **supportive bond** through regular phone calls, home visits, or specialized perinatal or pediatric bereavement discussion groups.

Grief is a process of ups and downs. Certain periods, such as the anniversary of a child's birth or death, or family celebrations, can intensify the pain. That's why it's essential to be attentive to these moments and to offer increased support during these stages. Families may need tools to commemorate these dates in a positive way, finding ways to continue honoring the child's memory while living with his or her absence.

## Helping to restore meaning and reconstruction

Grieving the loss of a child is never "complete", but it is possible, over time, to find a new way of living with the loss. One of the key roles of caregivers is to help parents **restore meaning** to their lives after the death. This may involve encouraging them to join bereavement support associations, to get involved in projects that pay tribute to their child, or simply to gradually rediscover activities that bring them comfort and joy.

Parents who lose a child may also need support to rebuild their relationship as a couple, which is often put to the test by bereavement. Each parent experiences loss in a different way, and this can sometimes create tensions or misunderstandings within the couple. Psychologists and caregivers can help them through these difficulties by offering them opportunities for dialogue and tools to help them better understand each other during this ordeal.

Finally, it's essential to recognize that the grieving process takes time, and that each family moves at its own pace. There is no "solution" to grief, but with the right support, families can learn to live with loss, honor their child's memory and rebuild a life where, despite absence, love and memories continue to give meaning.

# 13.

# Innovations and new technologies to support disabled children

- **New technologies for alternative communication (tablets, applications)**

**New technologies** are playing an increasingly crucial role in supporting children with disabilities, particularly when it comes to **alternative communication**. For children with communication difficulties, such as those with motor disabilities, autism spectrum disorders (ASD), language disorders or intellectual disabilities, tablets and dedicated applications offer effective, personalized solutions for expressing their needs and emotions, and interacting with their environment. These tools enable children to overcome barriers linked to speech or writing, thus promoting their social inclusion, autonomy and emotional well-being.

## The role of technology in alternative communication

Children who have difficulty communicating verbally can experience significant frustration, particularly when they are unable to express their needs or make themselves understood by those around them. This can lead to withdrawal or frustration-related crises. **Alternative communication technologies bridge this gap** by offering more accessible ways of expressing themselves, whether through images, pictograms, symbols, gestures or text. They enable children to regain a form of autonomy and interact more easily with their family, educational and social environment.

Tablets, with **adapted applications**, enable children to select images or words that translate what they want to say. These applications, often simple and intuitive, are designed to be easily manipulated, even by children with motor difficulties. Thanks to customizable interfaces, each child can have a communication system that matches his or her abilities and needs. For example, a child who is unable to speak can use an application that enables him or her to select pictograms representing objects, actions or emotions, which a voice synthesizer then enunciates for him or her.

# The advantages of tablets and applications for alternative communication

**Tablets** and **specialized applications** offer many advantages for alternative communication. First and foremost, they are **portable** and easy to handle, enabling children to take them everywhere, whether at school, at home or in public places. These tools thus facilitate integration into a variety of environments, without the child being limited by his or her communication difficulties.

One of the main advantages of these technologies is **their** ability to **adapt to the individual needs** of each child. Applications can be customized according to the child's level of development, type of disability and preferences. For example, some applications allow you to set specific images (family photos, familiar objects) or create pre-recorded phrases, while others offer a more complex choice of words and symbols for more advanced children. This flexibility makes communication more fluid and natural for the child.

In addition, the use of **voice synthesizers** integrated into these applications is a particularly powerful tool for non-verbal children. These synthesizers give the child a voice, by enunciating selected words or phrases. This not only facilitates communication with peers, but also boosts the child's self-esteem, as his or her message is taken into account and understood.

# Examples of applications for alternative communication

Today, there are several applications specifically designed to help children with communication difficulties. Among the most popular are :

- **Proloquo2Go**: A widely used application for children with language disorders. It features symbols and pictograms that the child can select to express needs or ideas. It is highly customizable and offers great flexibility to adapt to different skill levels.

- **Avaz**: This application is designed for children with speech disorders, particularly those with autism. It features an image- and text-based system, and can be used to initiate simple or complex conversations.

- **CoughDrop**: An online tool accessible via tablet or computer, enabling children to construct sentences by selecting symbols or words. It offers customization options adapted to the child's evolving skills.

- **LAMP Words for Life**: Specifically designed for children with ASD, LAMP uses an icon-based approach to encourage functional use of communication and stimulate language development.

These applications all offer **clear visual interfaces**, making them accessible even to children with cognitive or motor difficulties. They enable them to express themselves without necessarily using writing or speech, two skills that may be inaccessible to these children.

## The importance of support in the use of technology

Although **alternative communication technologies** offer immense potential, they require **support** to be fully effective. It is essential that professionals, whether speech therapists, specialized educators or caregivers, work closely with families to ensure that these tools are well integrated into the child's daily life. Initial training for the child and those around him is often necessary to learn how to use the applications optimally, and to adapt them to the child's changing needs.

Families also play a key role in the success of these tools, by using them regularly and creating a **stimulating communication environment**. For example, parents can encourage the child to use the tablet to express daily wishes (asking for a drink, expressing a desire to play) and to participate actively in family interactions. This helps to integrate technology into everyday life and strengthen the child's communication skills.

Finally, it is important to regularly monitor the **child's development** and ensure that the technology used is always adapted to his or her needs. Children with disabilities may progress in their development or encounter new challenges, which may require adjustments to technological tools.

## The challenges of using technology

Despite their many advantages, using new technologies for alternative communication presents certain **challenges**. Firstly, technological tools can be expensive, and not all families have access to the resources needed to acquire these tablets and applications. Public or private funding, as well as specialized associations, can play a role in making these tools available to children who need them most.

In addition, although technologies offer many possibilities, they should not replace **human interaction**. Technologies should be seen as a complement to other methods of communication, not as a total replacement. It is important to maintain an emotional and relational bond with the child, by combining the use of technology with direct interaction, games and moments of exchange.

- **Medical equipment and technical aids: wheelchairs, orthoses, etc.**

**Medical equipment** and **technical aids**, such as wheelchairs, orthoses and other devices, play a fundamental role in supporting children with disabilities. They help to compensate for physical limitations, promote autonomy, improve comfort and prevent medical complications. They are essential for improving children's quality of life and enabling them to participate in a wide range of social, educational and family activities. These devices are designed to adapt to the specific needs of each child, according to his or her type of disability and motor skills.

## Wheelchairs: mobility and independence

**Wheelchairs** are among the most commonly used technical aids for children with motor disorders or reduced mobility. They are essential to enable these children to move around independently, or with the assistance of family and friends. Wheelchairs can be **manual** or **electric**, depending on the child's degree of autonomy.

1. **Manual wheelchairs**: These wheelchairs are propelled by the user themselves or by a caregiver. They are often used by children who have sufficient arm strength to get around on their own, or by those whose relatives can push them. These wheelchairs are generally lighter, easier to transport and adapted to the needs of children with partial or total mobility of the lower limbs, but the ability to use the upper limbs.

2. **Electric wheelchairs**: These devices are motorized and enable the child to move around independently using a joystick or other adapted controls. They are suitable for children with more severe motor impairments, who are unable to move around in a manual wheelchair. Electric wheelchairs often feature sophisticated adjustments to adapt to the child's growth and changing needs. They are

designed to offer maximum comfort and autonomy, while taking into account limited motor skills.

Wheelchairs must be **customized** to suit the child. This includes adjustments to the seat, armrests, headrests and footrests to ensure good postural support, prevent pain associated with poor posture and reduce the risk of bedsores. Lighter, more easily foldable models also make life easier for families, particularly when travelling by car or public transport.

## Orthotics: correction and support

**Orthotics** are medical devices that help to correct or support a body part affected by a handicap or deficiency. They are widely used for children with motor, neuromuscular or orthopedic disorders, and are designed to **maintain, improve or restore** the function of a limb. These devices are often prescribed to improve posture, correct deformities, or prevent deformation of bones and joints.

1.  **Lower-limb orthoses**: These are devices that fit around the legs and feet to stabilize limbs and improve mobility. For example, children with cerebral palsy may need **orthopedic shoes** or **knee braces** to correct a deformity and improve their ability to walk. **Ankle-foot** splints are also commonly used to improve foot and leg alignment and aid walking.

2.  **Upper limb orthoses**: These may include **wrist splints** or **hand orthoses for** children who have difficulty using their arms or hands. These devices may be essential to improve grip function or to stabilize the upper limbs during daily activities. For example, a child with nerve damage in the arm may wear a brace to correct posture and strengthen the ability to use the arm as much as possible.

3.  **Orthopedic corsets**: These are used to support the spine in children with back problems, such as scoliosis or other

spinal deformities. Corsets help maintain good posture, prevent worsening of the deformity and improve day-to-day comfort.

Orthotics must be **custom-made** and regularly adjusted as the child grows. Regular up-follow by specialized professionals, such as orthoprosthetists and physiotherapists, is necessary to ensure that orthoses are adapted to the child's changing body and needs.

## Other technical aids: standing aids, walkers, etc.

In addition to wheelchairs and orthoses, there are many other devices to help disabled children **achieve mobility, comfort and independence**.

1.  **Standing** frames: These are devices designed to help children stand and adopt an upright position, even if they are unable to stand up on their own. Standing up has many health benefits: it improves blood circulation, prevents contractures, strengthens bones and aids digestion. Standing frames are often used for rehabilitation purposes, or for children who spend much of their time in a wheelchair. They enable the child to remain active, even in a standing position, by stimulating muscles and joints.

2.  **Walkers and** walking **frames**: These are designed for children who can walk but need extra support to maintain their balance. Walkers are often used for children with poor muscle strength or coordination. They enable them to move around safely, while working on their gross motor skills. They can be fitted with castors to facilitate movement, or with brakes to prevent falls.

3.  **Molded seats and specialized seating devices**: These devices are used to improve the posture of children who have difficulty maintaining a correct sitting position. They can be integrated into wheelchairs or used separately at home or at school. A custom-molded seat provides good

trunk and head support, improving comfort and preventing postural complications.

4. **Stairlifts and ramps**: These technical aids are particularly useful for facilitating movement in domestic or school environments. They enable children in wheelchairs or with reduced mobility to overcome architectural obstacles and access spaces they would not otherwise be able to access. Portable ramps are a quick and efficient solution, while stairlifts are more permanent and suitable for use in the home.

## The role of professionals in prescribing and monitoring equipment

Medical equipment and technical aids must be **prescribed** and **monitored** by qualified professionals, such as **rehabilitation physicians**, **occupational therapists** and **orthoprosthetists**. These professionals assess the child's needs according to his or her disability, level of development and daily environment. They take into account the **child's growth**, as equipment needs to be regularly adjusted or replaced to remain effective.

A proper assessment enables the most suitable equipment to be chosen, taking into account not only the medical aspects, but also the preferences and lifestyle of the child and his or her family. The role of the occupational therapist is particularly important in ensuring that the equipment fits in well with daily life, and enables the child to carry out the activities he or she wishes, whether at school, at home, or in leisure activities.

**Regular monitoring** is crucial to adjusting equipment to the child's changing needs, and to preventing complications arising from misuse or wear and tear. This may involve technical readjustments, repairs or even the replacement of certain parts of the equipment.

- **Virtual and augmented reality tools for sensory and cognitive rehabilitation**

**Virtual reality (VR)** and **augmented reality (AR) tools are** opening up new perspectives in **sensory and cognitive rehabilitation**, particularly for children with disabilities. These innovative technologies enable the creation of immersive, interactive environments that promote learning, sensory stimulation, cognitive recovery and the development of motor skills, while offering engaging, personalized experiences. Thanks to their flexibility and adaptability, these tools are used in a wide range of therapies to meet the specific needs of children with neurodevelopmental, motor or sensory disorders.

## What is virtual and augmented reality?

- **Virtual reality (VR)**: Virtual reality immerses users in a fully immersive, three-dimensional (3D) digital environment, where they can interact with virtual objects and spaces. Using a VR headset, children can immerse themselves in an environment specifically designed to stimulate certain skills, such as coordination, visual perception and memory.

- **Augmented reality (AR)**: Unlike VR, augmented reality adds digital elements to the real environment. Using tablets or smartphones, children can see virtual objects superimposed on the physical world, enriching their sensory and cognitive experience. AR is often more accessible than VR, as it doesn't require a headset and can be used in everyday contexts, such as in the classroom or at home.

## The benefits of VR and AR for sensory rehabilitation

Children with sensory deficits, such as vision, hearing or sensory integration disorders, can benefit from virtual and augmented reality technologies to enhance their perception and interaction with the world around them. These tools can simulate **rich**, controlled **sensory environments**, gradually stimulating the various senses and helping children to adapt to complex situations.

1. **Visual and auditory stimulation**: Virtual reality can recreate environments where visual or auditory perception is progressively stimulated. For example, interactive games in a VR environment can help a child to practice recognizing shapes, colors and movements, or to focus on specific sounds in an immersive and stimulating context. Auditory perception exercises, such as identifying sounds in a virtual room, can also be used for children with mild hearing difficulties.

2. **Sensory integration**: Children with **sensory integration disorders** may have difficulty processing and organizing sensory information from their environment. Virtual reality offers a controlled environment in which therapists can modulate the number of sensory stimuli, enabling the child to practice integrating different information (visual, auditory, tactile) at his or her own pace. For example, a child can be immersed in a virtual environment where he or she must touch objects while listening to instructions, thus integrating visual and auditory stimuli in a coordinated fashion.

3. **Proprioceptive and motor rehabilitation**: As part of motor rehabilitation, virtual reality can be used to help children improve their body awareness and perception of space. For example, VR games can encourage children to make specific movements to reach virtual objects, enabling them to develop proprioception - the perception of their own body's position and movement in space.

# The cognitive benefits of virtual and augmented reality tools

**Cognitive re-education** using VR and AR enables us to work on key functions such as **memory**, **attention**, **language** and **planning**. These tools are particularly beneficial for children with neurodevelopmental disorders, such as autism spectrum disorders (ASD), attention deficit disorder with or without hyperactivity (ADHD), or learning disabilities. Thanks to the interactivity and personalization offered by these technologies, cognitive exercises can be tailored to the specific needs of each child.

1. **Improving memory and attention**: VR and AR offer interactive games that stimulate memory and attention in a playful way. For example, a child can be immersed in a virtual environment where he or she must explore a city and memorize the location of objects or follow a sequence of instructions. These environments are designed to boost attention and concentration by stimulating different cognitive areas, without the child feeling that he or she is following a formal exercise.

2. **Development of executive functions**: Executive functions, such as planning, decision-making and problem-solving, are often impaired in children with neurodevelopmental disorders. AR or VR applications can simulate everyday tasks, such as shopping or preparing a virtual meal. These immersive games enable children to work on action planning, problem solving and time management, all while having fun.

3. **Working on communication and social interaction**: Children with communication disorders, including autistic children, can use VR to practice interacting in simulated social situations. For example, they can participate in virtual scenarios that reproduce everyday situations, such as going to school or chatting with peers. These controlled environments enable children to practice social interaction

without the anxiety-inducing aspects of the real world. AR, meanwhile, can enrich role-playing games or communication scenarios with visual elements that help reinforce the child's understanding and engagement.

## Practical applications of virtual and augmented reality in rehabilitation

Numerous **VR and AR applications** and **software** are already being used in sensory and cognitive rehabilitation. Practical examples include :

1.  **"MindMaze"**: a neurocognitive rehabilitation platform based on virtual reality. It is used to help children with brain injuries or cognitive disorders improve their motor and cognitive skills through interactive games.

2.  **"Jintronix"**: A motor rehabilitation program based on virtual reality, enabling children to carry out rehabilitation exercises at home, while being monitored remotely by healthcare professionals. Children can immerse themselves in playful environments, such as playing ball games or exploring virtual landscapes, while improving their coordination and mobility.

3.  **"Rehago"**: A virtual reality solution designed for rehabilitation after strokes, but also used for children suffering from cerebral palsy or other motor disorders. Children can practice fine and gross motor skills in a 3D environment.

4.  **"CoSpaces"**: An augmented reality application that lets children create their own interactive environments, stimulating both their cognitive skills (planning, problem-solving) and their creativity.

5.  **"VIRTUES"**: A virtual reality program designed to improve social skills in children with autism spectrum

disorders. It offers interactive virtual scenarios where the child can practice social behaviors and communication skills in a non-judgmental setting.

## The importance of support and limitations

Although VR and AR tools offer exceptional opportunities for rehabilitation, their **effectiveness depends largely on professional support**. Therapists, whether psychomotor therapists, speech therapists or occupational therapists, must supervise the use of these technologies to ensure that programs and virtual environments are adapted to the child's abilities and therapeutic goals. Personalization of exercises is often necessary to ensure that children progress at their own pace and are not overwhelmed by virtual stimuli.

However, it's also important to consider certain **limitations**. Some children may be sensitive to sensory overload, and immersive virtual environments need to be carefully modulated to avoid over-stimulation. What's more, the affordability of these tools can be an obstacle for some families, although public initiatives or subsidies exist to facilitate access to these technologies.

- **Integrating assistance and therapy robots into day-to-day care**

The integration of **assistance** and **therapy robots** into daily care represents a major technological advance in the support of children with disabilities. These robots, designed to interact with patients, provide therapeutic support, or assist with everyday tasks, help to improve children's autonomy, stimulate their cognitive and social development, and relieve caregivers of their work. They are part of a complementary approach to traditional care, providing innovative tools that facilitate children's care, while making their daily lives more fun and interactive.

# Assistive robots: a support for autonomy

**Assistive robots** are designed to help children with motor or cognitive limitations to carry out everyday tasks that they cannot perform on their own. These robots help to improve their independence and quality of life by taking over certain essential functions, or by providing them with tools to interact with their environment.

1.  **Telepresence and mobility robots**: These robots are used to help children move around or interact with places or people at a distance. For example, children with severe motor impairments can use **telepresence robots** to participate in school or social activities from home, when they cannot be physically present. These robots, often equipped with a camera, screen and microphone, enable the child to attend a class, interact with peers or communicate with family or carers remotely. This helps maintain an important social link, especially for children isolated by their condition.

2.  **Mobility assistance robots**: Robots such as the **exoskeleton robot** enable children with motor disorders to walk or move around independently. These mechanical devices attach to the child's limbs and assist movement, building muscle strength and improving coordination. They are particularly useful for children with cerebral palsy or other mobility-limiting conditions. By helping them to walk, these robots not only promote independence, they also help to strengthen muscles, improve balance, and prevent medical complications associated with prolonged immobility.

3.  **Assistive robots for everyday tasks**: Some robots, such as **JACO** or **iARM**, are robotic arms designed to help children perform gestures they can't do on their own, such as eating, grasping objects, opening doors or brushing their teeth. These robots are controlled by adapted

interfaces, such as voice commands, joysticks or even eye movements, enabling children to remain active in their daily activities. By increasing their autonomy in these tasks, these robots reduce the child's dependence on caregivers, while enabling them to feel more in control of their environment.

## Therapy robots: emotional and cognitive support

**Therapy robots**, also known as social robots, are used to improve the emotional and social well-being of children with neurodevelopmental disorders, sensory impairments or autism spectrum disorders (ASD). These robots, programmed to interact in a gentle, playful way, become play partners or therapeutic assistants, contributing to learning and social interaction.

1. **Interactive robots for social stimulation**: **NAO** or **Milo**, for example, are humanoid robots specially designed to help autistic children develop their social skills. They are programmed to interact with the child, reproducing facial expressions, asking questions or proposing educational activities. These robots enable children to practice recognizing emotions, following instructions or engaging in simple conversations, in a non-threatening environment. Children with autism, who may have difficulty interacting with adults or human peers, often find robots a less intimidating partner, helping them to overcome some of their social difficulties.

2. **Robots for cognitive stimulation**: Some robots are programmed to promote **cognitive development** by offering playful exercises adapted to the child's abilities. For example, **Leka** is a spherical robot designed for children with developmental disorders or disabilities. It offers educational activities that stimulate cognition, such as light, sound and movement games, while encouraging social interaction and motor skills. This type of robot

helps children develop skills in problem-solving, hand-eye coordination and attention.

3.  **Emotional robots for emotional support**: Robots such as **PARO**, a seal-shaped robot, are used to provide emotional comfort to children who may be experiencing anxiety, stress or sadness. Thanks to their soft, soothing appearance, these robots offer emotional support by responding to petting and making reassuring sounds. They are particularly effective in situations where children are faced with anxiety-provoking medical procedures, or in palliative care. Interaction with these robots can help reduce stress and provide a sense of emotional security, particularly for children who find it difficult to verbalize their emotions.

## The benefits of integrating robots into the care sector

The integration of robots into care presents several **advantages** for disabled children and caregivers alike.

1.  **Enhanced autonomy**: Assistive robots enable children to acquire greater independence in their daily lives, whether in terms of mobility, domestic tasks or communication. By reducing their dependence on their parents or caregivers, these robots boost children's self-confidence and help them feel more involved in their own lives.

2.  **Social and cognitive stimulation**: therapy robots provide innovative solutions for encouraging children to interact, communicate and learn. Through playful, repetitive interactions, they help children to develop their social and cognitive skills in a progressive way, adapted to their abilities. Robots also provide an interesting alternative to conventional therapy methods, making rehabilitation sessions more motivating and engaging for children.

3. **Emotional support**: Children with disabilities are often confronted with high levels of stress, anxiety or frustration, particularly when they are unable to express their needs or interact with their environment smoothly. Robots, with their predictable responses and soothing behaviors, offer valuable emotional support. By enabling them to feel understood and accompanied, these devices improve their emotional well-being and reduce their anxiety.

4. **Reducing the burden on caregivers**: Parents and caregivers are often exhausted by the repetitive tasks and constant care required by children with disabilities. Assistive robots can alleviate this burden by taking over certain tasks, such as helping with mobility, eating or educational activities. This enables caregivers to concentrate more on emotional and relational support, rather than the purely functional aspects of care.

## The challenges of integrating robots into healthcare

Despite their many advantages, the use of robots in care also brings certain **challenges**. Firstly, **the high cost of** these technologies can be a barrier to some families or institutions, although public funding and assistance may be available. In addition, **training** caregivers and families in the use of these robots is essential to ensure their effectiveness. Robots often require customization and regular management to adapt to children's evolving needs.

Another challenge concerns the **emotional and social acceptance of** these robots by the children themselves. While some children quickly become attached to these devices, others may be reluctant to interact with a machine. Robots need to be gradually integrated into the child's daily life, taking care to respect his or her preferences and pace of adaptation.

- **Using technology for sensory stimulation and playful learning**

The use of **technologies for sensory stimulation** and **playful learning** offers exceptional opportunities for children with disabilities or special educational needs. These technologies make it possible to create immersive, engaging and interactive experiences that foster children's cognitive, motor and emotional development. By combining **sensory stimulation** and **learning through play**, they capture children's attention, boost their learning capacity and help them overcome challenges related to communication, motor skills and sensory regulation. Whether in the form of **interactive games**, **virtual or augmented realities**, or **educational applications**, technologies can be a powerful complement to more traditional learning methods.

## The importance of sensory stimulation

**Sensory stimulation** plays a crucial role in the development of children, especially those with developmental disorders or disabilities. It helps to develop and refine the child's ability to perceive, integrate and respond to sensory information from the environment. Children with **sensory integration disorders** may have difficulty processing sensory stimuli (noise, light, texture, movement), and adapted technologies can modulate these stimuli to make them more accessible and progressive.

1. **Visual stimulation**: Interactive games and applications using bright colors, lights and shapes stimulate children's vision. For example, shape or color recognition games help refine visual skills and discrimination of objects in the environment.

2. **Auditory stimulation**: Technologies can incorporate soft sounds, music or interactive stories to help children better perceive auditory sounds and nuances. For example, auditory sensory games can help children locate sounds, distinguish between different noises, or follow simple verbal instructions.

3.  **Tactile stimulation**: Children who need **tactile stimulation** can use tactile interfaces on tablets or devices that incorporate pressure sensors or textures. Apps allow them to play with virtual objects and experience sensory feedback, helping to develop their tactile perception and improve hand-eye coordination.

4.  **Proprioceptive and vestibular stimulation**: Games that incorporate movement (via interactive platforms or virtual reality devices) can improve balance, coordination and awareness of the body in space. For example, interactive games that encourage children to move or manipulate objects in virtual reality are a fun way to work on gross motor skills.

## Technologies for sensory stimulation: tools and devices

A variety of technological tools are specifically designed to provide **sensory stimulation** for children with special needs:

1.  **Interactive sensory rooms**: Rooms specially equipped with immersive technologies, such as projectors, interactive lights, sound effects and tactile surfaces. These rooms allow children to explore a stimuli-rich environment, where they can interact with lighted objects, listen to soothing sounds, or manipulate objects projected on the walls or floor. For example, systems such as **Snoezelen offer** soothing multi-sensory environments that help children relax and open up to stimuli they find difficult to integrate into their daily lives.

2.  **Touch tablets and sensory applications**: Many tablet applications are designed to offer engaging sensory experiences. Applications such as **Autism iHelp** or **Sensory Light Box** create interactive visual and auditory environments. Children can touch the screen to manipulate luminous objects, generate sounds or create visual effects

that stimulate several senses simultaneously. These applications enable the intensity of stimuli to be controlled, and can be customized according to the child's needs.

3.  **Virtual reality (VR) and augmented reality (AR)**: These technologies enable the creation of immersive **environments where** children can interact with virtual worlds specially designed to meet their sensory needs. For example, a virtual reality application could immerse a child in a quiet forest, where they can explore natural sounds, touch 3D visual elements, or simply relax in a soothing environment. These tools are particularly effective for children who have difficulty managing sensory stimuli in real environments.

4.  **Interactive robots**: Some **therapy robots**, such as **Leka** or **Paro**, are designed to provide sensory stimulation while encouraging social interaction. These robots emit sounds, vibrations or lights, and react to the child's touch, encouraging sensory engagement. Leka, for example, is a small, spherical, luminous robot that moves and interacts with the child according to the stimuli it receives, stimulating the visual, auditory and tactile senses in equal measure.

## Fun learning through technology

**Fun educational technologies** combine fun and learning. They transform the learning experience into an interactive game that captures the child's attention and enables them to become actively involved in their own development. Playful learning becomes particularly important for children with disabilities, as it overcomes some traditional barriers by making learning activities more accessible and motivating.

1. **Educational video games**: Many video games are designed to develop specific skills, such as logic, memory, problem-solving and communication. For example, games like "**Osmo**" combine real objects with digital interaction on a tablet, enabling children to manipulate shapes, letters or objects in a stimulating game that enhances their cognitive skills.

2. **Interactive applications for learning**: Applications such as **Khan Academy Kids, ABCmouse,** or **Endless** Alphabet transform learning into a series of fun challenges where the child must solve riddles, match objects, or follow instructions to progress. These applications are often visually attractive and rich in sound content, making them accessible to children with special needs. They also offer adjustable levels of difficulty, enabling each child to learn at his or her own pace.

3. **Augmented reality for learning**: **Augmented reality (AR)** enables virtual elements to be superimposed on real objects, offering a unique way of making learning more visual and interactive. For example, applications such as **Quiver** or **AR Flashcards** transform 2D images into 3D objects that children can manipulate and explore. This makes abstract concepts, such as mathematics or biology, more concrete and easier to understand.

4. **Virtual reality systems for learning**: Virtual reality can simulate interactive environments where children can explore worlds, solve puzzles or take part in immersive learning experiences. Programs such as **Virtual Reality Classrooms** and **Google Expeditions allow** children to travel virtually to museums, planets or ancient civilizations, stimulating their curiosity while developing their skills.

# The importance of personalization and support

For sensory stimulation and playful learning technologies to be effective, they need to be **tailored to** the specific needs of each child. Follow-up by **healthcare professionals**, such as occupational therapists, speech therapists or specialized educators, is essential to adapt these tools to the child's development, and to ensure that they meet precise therapeutic objectives.

Caregivers and educators also need to be trained in the use of these technologies, so that they can guide the child in their use and adjust settings according to his or her level of development. Regular supervision is important to ensure that technological tools remain motivating and beneficial to the child's learning, while avoiding sensory overload.

# 14.

# Recommendations for future caregivers in the pediatric field

- • **The essential qualities of a good pediatric orderly**

**The essential qualities of a good pediatric orderly** go far beyond mere technical competence. Working with children, particularly those who are ill or disabled, requires specific skills that are as much human as they are professional. Caregivers play a central role in the care of young patients: they are the first point of contact, offering them comfort, helping them with their daily routine and supporting their families during this often trying time. To be fully successful in this role, certain qualities are essential.

## Empathy and listening

One of the fundamental qualities of a good pediatric orderly is undoubtedly **empathy**. Indeed, working with sick children requires a great ability to understand their emotions, fears and needs, even when they are unable to express them clearly. Children, especially the very young, can be anxious about medical care, especially as they don't always understand what's happening to them. The caregiver needs to be able to **sense** these anxieties and bring them comfort, adapting his or her approach in a gentle and caring way.

**Listening** is also crucial in this context. It's not just a question of listening to what the child says, but also of being attentive to his non-verbal expressions: a look, a gesture, a change in attitude. Each sign can reveal what the child is feeling. For example, a child who refuses to eat or move may be expressing pain, discomfort or fear that he or she has not yet been able to verbalize. By listening attentively and understanding, the caregiver is often the one who alerts the nursing team to these subtle but crucial details, enabling them to adjust their care.

## Patience and gentleness

**Patience** is an essential quality when it comes to caring for children. Young patients, especially those with chronic illnesses or disabilities, can take a long time to adapt to care or to accept medical procedures. Sometimes, they are resistant or refractory to care, which can complicate the act of care. The caregiver must be patient, respect the child's rhythm and never be brusque or hasty, even in stressful situations. It can take a long time to gain a child's trust, but this patience pays off when it creates a climate of security and cooperation.

**Gentleness** is also essential in the approach to care. In addition to technical gestures, the caregiver must show delicacy in the way he or she speaks to and touches the child. A reassuring tone of voice, light, soothing gestures and a caring attitude can greatly reduce the stress felt by the young patient. This gentleness is particularly important during sensitive moments of care, such as body hygiene or the fitting of medical devices. The caregiver's gentleness humanizes care and creates a bond of trust with the child.

## Observation skills

A good pediatric orderly must also **have** a **keen sense of observation**. Children, especially the very young, are not always in a position to say exactly how they feel. The caregiver must therefore be able to detect subtle signs of discomfort, pain or unease. This may manifest itself in behavioral changes, refusal to eat, unusual restlessness or, on the contrary, excessive fatigue. By being attentive to these details, the caregiver plays a key role in detecting the first signs of complication or worsening of the patient's state of health, and can thus alert the nursing team to the need for more appropriate care.

## The ability to build trust

**Creating a bond of trust** with the child is essential if he or she is to accept care and feel secure. The caregiver's caring attitude often becomes a point of reference for the child, someone he or she can trust and turn to in times of need. This relationship is all the more important as children may be separated from their parents or family environment for extended periods. By establishing this trust, the caregiver helps the child to cope better with hospitalization or treatment.

This relationship of trust also extends to **parents**, who, at times of great anxiety, need to feel that their child is being cared for competently and humanely. The caregiver must know how to reassure parents, listen to them and offer moral support, while respecting their emotions and concerns. By being present at their side, they help to alleviate the psychological pressure they may feel.

## Versatility and adaptability

The day-to-day work of a pediatric orderly is highly varied and requires great **versatility**. Each child is unique and has specific needs, depending on age, illness or psychomotor development. Caregivers must therefore be able to adapt quickly to different situations, whether caring for a premature infant in neonatology, a child undergoing rehabilitation, or an adolescent suffering from a chronic illness. This ability to adapt also implies knowing how to adjust one's approach according to the reactions of each child, as certain care techniques are better accepted by one child than another.

In addition to this versatility in technical gestures, the caregiver must also demonstrate **emotional adaptability**. Pediatric care can be emotionally taxing, especially when confronted with a child's suffering or difficult situations such as the end of life. Caregivers need to know how to manage their own emotions, while remaining available and attentive, so that they can continue to provide quality care at what can sometimes be a very difficult time.

## A sense of responsibility and team spirit

In pediatrics, the caregiver is part of a **multidisciplinary team** made up of doctors, nurses, psychologists, physiotherapists and specialized educators. He/she must be able to work in collaboration with these different professionals, sharing the information necessary for the proper care of the child and respecting care protocols. A sense of **responsibility** is essential, as the caregiver is often the first to be in direct contact with the child. They must therefore be able to react quickly and effectively to any problems that may arise, while complying with the medical team's directives.

Team spirit also translates into **solidarity** between colleagues. Working in pediatrics can be physically and emotionally exhausting, and mutual support between team members is essential to maintaining a good standard of care and a healthy working environment. Regular exchanges and open communication help us to better understand the needs of our young patients, and to adjust collectively to meet them in the best possible way.

- **How to prepare for a career caring for children with disabilities**

Preparing for a career in the care of **children with disabilities** is a process that combines both technical training and personal commitment. This career requires specialized skills, a deep understanding of children's needs, and the human qualities essential to creating a caring and secure environment. Here are the main steps in preparing for this demanding but rewarding profession.

## 1. Acquire specialized training and technical skills

The first step in preparing for a career in caring for children with disabilities is to obtain solid professional training. Depending on the role you wish to play, there are several courses of study to consider, such as **care assistant**, **pediatric nurse**, **physiotherapist**, **occupational therapist** or **psychomotrician**.

- **State health diplomas**: Diplomas such as the **Diplôme d'État d'Aide-Soignant (DEAS)** or the **Diplôme d'État d'Infirmier (DEI)** are essential foundations for starting out in this field. These courses offer instruction in basic care, pain management, hygiene and overall care of the child. They can then be complemented by specializations in pediatrics or care of children with disabilities.

- **Specialized training in pediatrics and disability**: To better understand the particularities of children with disabilities, it is often recommended to follow specific modules dedicated to physical, sensory, cognitive and mental disabilities. These courses go into greater depth on how to adapt care, communication techniques and the use of assistive devices (wheelchairs, orthoses, alternative communication technologies, etc.).

- **Internships and professional practice**: In addition to theoretical training, it is essential to complete internships in specialized facilities, such as medical-social establishments, schools for disabled children or pediatric hospitals. These experiences enable you to discover the day-to-day care of children with disabilities, observe how professionals adapt their interventions, and develop practical skills in real-life contexts. These internships also provide an opportunity to gain a better understanding of multidisciplinary teamwork, which is essential in this career.

## 2. Developing essential human qualities

Beyond technical training, human qualities are crucial to success in this profession. Caring for handicapped children requires constant attention, empathy and a caring attitude to create a bond of trust with the child and his or her family.

- **Empathy and listening skills**: Children with disabilities, especially those who can't express themselves verbally, need a deep understanding of their situation and needs. It's essential to be able to put yourself in their shoes, feel their emotions and react appropriately to their signals, even when they are subtle. Listening to families is also crucial to providing appropriate support and alleviating their concerns.

- **Patience and gentleness**: Progress can be slow for some children, especially those with severe disabilities. Patience is therefore essential to support the child at his or her own pace, without becoming discouraged. Care gestures must be performed with great gentleness to avoid adding stress or discomfort. Gentleness also helps gain the child's trust, which is essential if he or she is to feel safe during care.

- **Adaptability**: Each child is unique and requires a personalized approach. The caregiver or nurse must adapt his or her interventions to the child's state of health, type of disability, abilities and emotional reactions. For example, the way you approach a child with autism will be different from the way you approach a child with a motor disability. This adaptability is essential to meet the specific needs of each child, while respecting his or her rhythm.

## 3. Understanding the different types of disability

To provide appropriate care, it is necessary to **understand the different types of disability** and their impact on children's daily lives.

- **Motor disabilities**: Children with motor disabilities, such as cerebral palsy, may need support with mobility, feeding or hygiene. Understanding how to adapt care to physical limitations, and using support devices such as wheelchairs or sit-to-stand devices, is fundamental to ensuring maximum autonomy.

- **Sensory disabilities**: Children with hearing or visual impairments require adaptations in communication and environment. For example, it may be necessary to learn **alternative communication** techniques, such as sign language or interactive visual tools, to better interact with them.

- **Cognitive and mental disabilities**: These disabilities, which include disorders such as autism, require a specific approach. It is essential to understand the social and behavioral challenges associated with these disorders, as well as the support methods that can help develop these children's cognitive and social skills, while reducing their anxiety.

## 4. Mastering assistance tools and technologies

Working with disabled children often involves the use of specific **technologies and technical aids**. Familiarity with these tools is essential for effective and appropriate care.

- **Mobility tools**: Devices such as wheelchairs, walkers or exoskeletons help children to move around and participate in activities. It's important to know how to adjust these devices to ensure your child's safety and comfort.

- **Alternative communication technologies**: Many disabled children have difficulty expressing themselves verbally. It is therefore essential to master technologies such as **communication tablets**, pictograms or Makaton language, which enable children to communicate their needs and emotions non-verbally.

- **Rehabilitation aids**: Some children require functional rehabilitation sessions. The use of re-education devices, sensory stimulation software or interactive robots can help children progress in their motor or cognitive development, in a fun and adapted way.

# 5. Working in a multidisciplinary team

Caring for children with disabilities is rarely an individual mission. It requires **teamwork** with a variety of professionals: doctors, physiotherapists, occupational therapists, psychologists, specialized educators, and so on. It is therefore essential to develop the ability to collaborate with these professionals, share information and coordinate care. This multidisciplinary approach ensures comprehensive care for the child, taking into account his or her physical, psychological and social needs.

The **exchange of information** between professionals is crucial to guaranteeing continuity of care and adjusting interventions according to the child's progress or difficulties. For example, a caregiver may alert the team to a change in the child's behavior or health, enabling a reassessment of care.

- **The importance of resilience and adaptability**

**Resilience** and **adaptability** are essential qualities, particularly in professions related to the care of children with disabilities. They enable professionals to overcome daily challenges, adjust to children's changing needs, and preserve their own well-being in the face of often demanding situations. These two qualities complement each other and are essential to providing quality support for both the child and his or her family.

# Resilience: coping with emotional and professional challenges

**Resilience** is the ability to bounce back from difficulties, recover from stressful situations and maintain a positive attitude despite obstacles. In the field of caring for children with disabilities, resilience is paramount, as caregivers are regularly confronted with emotionally complex situations.

1. **Dealing with emotional exhaustion**: Working with disabled children often involves witnessing moments of suffering or frustration. Children may face chronic pain, learning difficulties or developmental delays that require constant attention and support. Resilience enables caregivers to continue to offer quality care, even when faced with these difficult moments, by striking a balance between empathy for the child and managing their own emotional load.

2. **Maintaining motivation**: Progress in children with disabilities can be slow or irregular. Caregivers may face periods when progress is minimal or non-existent. Resilience enables them to persevere, to remain motivated and committed despite obstacles, and to rejoice in small victories, even if they are not always immediately visible. It's a key quality for avoiding discouragement and continuing to believe in each child's ability to progress, at his or her own pace.

3. **Supporting families**: Parents of disabled children often go through periods of discouragement, sadness or exhaustion. Caregivers' resilience plays an important role in the support they can provide to families, offering attentive listening, reassurance and advice on how to manage difficult times. By being able to stay strong and maintain a positive attitude, caregivers become a beacon for parents on their own emotional journey.

## Adaptability: adjusting care to changing needs

**Adaptability** is the ability to adjust to changes, to modulate interventions according to new or unforeseen situations. It's an indispensable quality in the care of children with disabilities, where needs can evolve rapidly and each child presents particularities that require a personalized approach.

1.  **Adapting to individual needs**: Every child with a disability has specific needs, which may vary according to his or her physical, cognitive or emotional condition. An adaptable caregiver knows how to adjust his or her approach to meet these needs, by modifying care techniques, the way of communicating, or even adapting to the child's reactions. For example, an autistic child may require non-verbal communication techniques, while a child with a motor disability may need specific mobility support.

2.  **Reacting to unforeseen situations**: Children with disabilities may face sudden complications or changes in their health status that require rapid adjustments. Adaptability enables the caregiver to respond effectively to these unforeseen situations, whether by modifying a care plan, collaborating with the care team to find a solution, or reassuring the child and family.

3.  **Accompanying life transitions**: Children with disabilities often go through transitional stages, whether it's starting school, adapting to a new medical device, or changes in their treatment. Adaptability is crucial to accompanying these transitions smoothly, supporting the child through these new stages and adjusting interventions to meet emerging needs. This also includes the ability to work as part of a team with other professionals (special educators, physiotherapists, etc.) to offer comprehensive, coordinated support.

## Combining resilience and adaptability in care

By combining **resilience** and **adaptability**, caregivers can respond effectively to the emotional and technical demands of their profession. These qualities enable them not only to overcome challenges, but also to support children and their families in an ever-changing care environment.

**Resilience** enables caregivers to cope with emotional challenges without becoming overwhelmed, while **adaptability** gives them the flexibility to adjust care to the child's changing needs. Together, these qualities help create a climate of trust, caring and ongoing support, where each child is cared for with respect for his or her individuality and specific needs.